Praise for *Awakenin*

"This book makes me very happy. First, as a woman, it is ~~~
to read the work of a man who is devoted to the wisdom and transformative power
of the divine feminine. As a psychiatrist, it is immeasurably helpful to have a clear
framework to understand the gift of the extraordinary consciousness beyond
our usual body-mind perspective. Understanding the creative process of Shakti's
unfolding in the evolution of our Self is a much-needed perspective in interpreting
the physical, mental, and emotional challenges that can arise in us—whether or
not we are actively seeking to cultivate the vital flow of Kundalini. Dr. Edwards
provides detailed guidance for exploring meditative techniques and other tools
to work with this ancient tradition in our everyday lives. Further, he provides a
balanced treatment of the psychological process encountered in inner work,
including the healthful role of the ego mind and working with our shadow in the
process of Kundalini awakening—essential but often neglected topics in spiritual
guidance. This is an inspiring reference manual for my work with others."

MARY B. O'MALLEY, MD, PHD

"This book is a revelation that is a service to all of us—beginner, initiate, sage. It
is a book about awakening that inspires awakening. It is a book about honoring
the feminine that is a true sacred marriage of the masculine and feminine—
remarkably clear and beautifully poetic. The book is elegant in the truest scientific
and consciousness-based ways—simple and so powerful. Lawrence Edwards
supportively guides us on our own heroic journey in a way that demonstrates he is
what he writes about—so humble and so wise. A real teacher."

ANDREW HAHN, PSYD
Founder and director of the Guided Self Healing Training Institute

"This book is an indispensable guide for anyone on the path of spiritual awakening.
Dr. Edwards has devoted his life to studying and practicing the unfolding process
of Kundalini, the subtle spiritual energy within everyone that leads to the highest
states of consciousness. His depth of knowledge, personal experiences, and
devotional poems illuminate the pages of this extraordinary book. Acknowledged
worldwide for his professional experience in guiding people along the spiritual
path—particularly through the mysteries of advanced yogic practice—Dr. Edwards
is a gifted and compassionate guide. His devotional journey will inspire all who
read his book. It is destined to become a classic in the field."

OLIVIA AMES HOBLITZELLE
Author of *Ten Thousand Joys & Ten Thousand Sorrows: A Couple's Journey through Alzheimer's*

"A rare combination of a highly trained, articulate Western mind and a deeply personal experience of this extraordinary subject. Wise, elegant, and inspiring. Highly recommended."

LEE LYON

Founder and director of the Foundation for Integrative Meditation

"Lawrence Edwards has given us an incomparable gift: a detailed, compassionate, and brilliantly clear guide to the greatest mystery and greatest revelation of our existence. It tells the story of his call to the profound process of awakening known in the yogic tradition as Kundalini, through his early visionary experiences, his meeting with his Indian teacher, Swami Muktananda, and how his life unfolded from that fortuitous meeting. Drawing on the rich legacy of numerous traditions—Jungian, Western psychology, scientific research, traditional yogic and mystical ones—this book is an incomparable aid in taking us beyond the confines of the delusionary certainties of our ego mind toward the experience of the deepest ground of our own being. Kundalini—known by other names in other spiritual traditions—is the path of reunion with the Divine Consciousness that lives and breathes in all of us—capable, as he says, of transforming our mind, our body, and every aspect of our lives. There is no one better qualified to explain and teach it, or to accompany us on our own mythic journey of discovery."

ANNE BARING

Author of *The Dream of the Cosmos: A Quest for the Soul*

"This book is 'state of the art'—the most comprehensive discussion of the Universal Life Force known as Kundalini. Edwards explores spiritual principles with his unique expertise in psychology, neuroscience, meditation training, and spiritual traditions. Western psychology has mapped our psychological and emotional development. Western medicine has mapped our physical development. Now Edwards shows us, in unprecedented depth, each step of our spiritual development. Toward the end of this excellent read, Edwards helps us to experience the realization that we humans are capable of and entitled to the wonder and splendor of each moment."

CHARLES L. WHITFIELD, MD

Author of *Choosing God: A Bird's Eye View of a Course in Miracles,* and

BARBARA H. WHITFIELD, RT

Author of *Spiritual Awakenings: Insights of the Near-Death Experience and other Doorways to Our Soul*

AWAKENING
KUNDALINI

AWAKENING KUNDALINI

the path to radical freedom

Lawrence Edwards, PhD

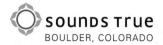

SOUNDS TRUE
BOULDER, COLORADO

Sounds True, Inc.
Boulder, CO 80306

All names used throughout the book have been changed to protect patients' privacy.

Published 2013

Cover and book design by Karen Polaski
Cover photo © Shooter from Shutterstock.com

Printed in the United States of America

Library of Congress Cataloging-in-Publication Data
Edwards, Lawrence, Ph. D.
  Awakening kundalini : the path to radical freedom / Lawrence Edwards, PhD.
     pages cm
Includes bibliographical references.
ISBN 978-1-60407-932-6
1. Kundalini. I. Title.
BL1238.56.K86E39 2013
204'.36—dc23
              2013010783

Ebook ISBN: 978-1-62203-066-8

10 9 8 7 6 5 4 3 2 1

Shree Kundalini
Invocation

O Kundalini Devi,
though known by a thousand names
no one can merely summon you.
Yet, the scent of love from sweet ripe souls
instantly draws you near!

Dancing as bliss,
casting off sparks of infinite delight,
you set souls ablaze!
Ignite us like a torch
my Beloved!
Throw the sodden logs of mind and body
onto your conflagration of Love!
Release the light and life
hidden within us!

O my Beloved,
whether clothed in form
or moving through the universe unseen,
graceful Holy Spirit,
protector of lovers of the Divine,
You are inseparable
from the eternal One.

Embracing all seekers wandering the worlds
You usher them home
to delight in true freedom.
May we be worthy of your
boundless love and protection.

O my Beloved Kundalini,
awaken seekers to your sublime play
of hide and seek!
There's nothing You can't create!
You take forms that delude or enlighten,
lead us astray or draw us into your arms.
Delivering the fruits of our choices,
refining our discrimination,
You reveal the power you've given us
to create every reality.
Grant that we remain ever vigilant
of the power we wield
and guide us to use it only
in the service of love and compassion.

Plucking a strand of light from your countenance,
even as it forever vibrates with Om,
You string luminous jewels of consciousness
upon this thread
and spin a multi-colored shimmering web
of mind and body around it.
There You are,
throbbing within us,
piercing the veils,
inviting us to follow your love call!
May we remain true to even the subtlest
sounds of your voice.

You've taken the form of the bindu,
exalted portal shrouded in mystery,
confounding all but those empty of self.

Carry us through your gateway to the Infinite,
known only through union with You.

In your earthly domain
You embrace your Beloved.
Taking the ancient,
yet ever-new serpentine form,
You coil round Him in pure delight!

In your transcendent abode
You both disappear!
No one can say
where Lover and Beloved have gone!

You are the path of Love,
You reveal the power of devotion
and take the form of its fruits,
nourishing your seeking-self.
Give us the wisdom
to take refuge in You alone.

Your inexhaustible Light illumines our path,
freeing us from all pain born of your ignorance.
You become sounds and mantras,
words and scriptures,
gods and goddesses
out of your boundless compassion
and unfathomable yearning to set us free.
What won't you become
to meet your seekers' needs?
What won't You give of yourself
to ease our way to freedom?
Your generosity humbles us.
Please open our hearts to all!

O my Beloved,
There's nothing you won't reveal

to the wise soul humbled by knowing
their afflictions.
Mother of the universe,
by Your grace I now see
all forms are Your form.
Regardless of how You appear in the moment,
enemy or friend,
wise or foolish,
let me worship You
with offerings of loving kindness,
joy and delight.

O Beloved Kundalini,
adored form of Ma Kali,
You illumine her darkest mysteries!
Dwelling in the hearts of all my dearest,
I bow to You.

O graceful Lady of Light,
release me from the bonds of suffering,
extinguish all cravings
save the one for You.
I beg You my Beloved,
let me serve You
until all are free.

OFFERED BY KALIDAS
October 2013
Inspired by the Kundalini Stavaha[1]

Contents

Preface

f someone were to pick up a rock, put it in your hand, and ask you if it was real or not, you'd likely say, "yes, it is real!" without hesitation and probably wonder why a person would ask such a question. The ordinary mind, our ego mind, is almost always certain that it knows and understands basic reality—but being so convinced that we know something, as unconscious and unintentional as that attitude may be, makes us blind to all that we don't know. Holding on to that rock, the ordinary mind has no sense that the stone is 99.99 percent empty space, and what is perceived as a rock is actually pure energy bound in that form! The same can be said of the one holding it.

Cutting through the blindness of the ordinary mind, cutting through ignorance and the pride-of-knowing delusion, requires a force of wisdom beyond the closed mind's tangle of ideas and beliefs. Cutting through the mind allows us to directly know the highest truths. One term for that force of wisdom and ultimate knowing is *Kundalini*. Kundalini is a Sanskrit yogic term for the unimpeded power of wisdom, transformation, and revelation inherent to us all. It is the power of universal, unbounded Consciousness as the potential for the individual to know all that lies beyond the confines of the mind and body while discovering a new vision of the mind and body revealing hidden dimensions with unimagined clarity.

The term *Kundalini* translates quite literally as "the coiled one" and symbolically points to our innate potential power of consciousness, which is represented by a coiled spring or a snake, ready to be unleashed. The unfurling of Kundalini's power occurs through the process of Kundalini awakening, which releases the power of Infinite Consciousness to impact the mind and body in countless transformative ways. It unleashes the power and potential of your mind and body to function at their very best. More importantly, from a yogic perspective, this power, your power, opens experiences of boundless love, compassion, wisdom, and grace. Ultimately Kundalini brings you to the highest state of consciousness possible.

The aim of this book is to support people on their path of spiritual awakening, regardless of the tradition they follow. Kundalini is given different names in different spiritual traditions—Holy Spirit, Chi, Sophia, N'um, Saraswati, Tara, Prajnaparamita, bodhicitta, and many more—but the power of grace, revelation, and transformation to which these terms point is one and the same. Each language has its name for gold, but gold is always the same substance. All spiritual traditions speak of the power beyond the mind that draws one through the profound process of transformation and revelation to the very source of the highest wisdom and boundless love. That power, in the yogic tradition, is known as Kundalini.

Kundalini's Quest

The Full Embrace of Life

> It would not be too much to say that myth is the secret
> opening through which the inexhaustible energies of
> the cosmos pour into human cultural manifestation.
>
> JOSEPH CAMPBELL[1]

As I hear from individuals around the world about their Kundalini stirrings and awakenings, I am struck by the enormous variety of contexts in which these experiences occur. Kundalini shows her sometimes fierce, other times gentle, and always loving face in the personal transformations and awakenings that occur through yoga practices, religious practices, chanting and mantra practices, through trauma and near-death experiences, during sex, in intense prayer, in the violence of war, while out in nature, and in countless other ways. Kundalini can even begin to move when you are doing absolutely nothing in particular.

For decades I've had the extreme good fortune to live a life embraced by Kundalini and dedicated to Kundalini. By following her path, serving and studying under great teachers, and offering the *seva* (selfless service) of mentoring people moving through Kundalini's labyrinth, every aspect of my life has been touched by her grace. I was drawn to Kundalini because of profoundly transformative experiences that occurred sometimes spontaneously and at other times while doing structured meditation and yoga practices.

For the last several years, I've been the head of the Kundalini Research Network, lecturing at conferences, teaching, and encountering people from all walks of life who have been touched by Kundalini. In the yogic tradition, Kundalini is described as "ever new," and now, almost forty-five years since I first heard of Kundalini, She remains as fascinating, fresh, and grace-filled as ever. She is the eternal dancer beckoning us to awaken to the boundless delight of her dance.

From the most expansive perspective of the macrocosm, Kundalini is Shakti, the infinite power of Consciousness that creates the entire universe and everything within it. From an interior, microcosmic perspective, Kundalini creates the universe of body and mind, every cell and every thought, while holding the potential power to directly know what is completely beyond the mind, beyond words, beyond even the imagination. These kinds of self-transcendent experiences, transpersonal in nature, can unfold over time and profoundly impact our lives. Transpersonal experiences come in many ways; they can happen in dreams, in sudden experiences walking down the street, in the midst of nature, or as one woman told me, in the Walmart parking lot! They aren't all Kundalini-related in the classic yogic sense, but they all reflect our innate power to perceive, to get glimpses of what lies beyond the curtain that marks the boundary of the ordinary mind.

We naturally possess the capability of consciousness to suddenly or progressively go beyond the ordinary confines of the mind-body-self. We all have the ability to experience how transcendent Consciousness can illumine things that the ordinary mind finds quite extraordinary. That's really what is at the heart of understanding Kundalini as the power of Universal Consciousness. Kundalini is the power of transformation through illumination, revelation, and energetic re-creation of the mind-body vehicle. It is the motive power of every mystical/ spiritual tradition, though each calls it by a different name.

It's the birthright of every human being to know Kundalini and through this power of grace, to know the Divine as Self. It's *your* innate capacity. The term *Kundalini* may sound foreign, but the power itself is as near to you as your breath. It's closer to you than any thought; it throbs within you more deeply than your beating heart. It's present in every aspect of your life.

I'm regularly contacted by people with unrecognized stirrings of Kundalini's powers. Many of these people are engaged in intense spiritual practices from traditions not typically thought of as Kundalini-related, while on a Tibetan or Zen Buddhist retreat, for example, or while practicing centering prayer or shamanic rituals. Kundalini experiences begin for some individuals after surviving terrorist attacks or battle injuries. Some people have had awakening experiences while in the process of recovery from addictions. And still others simply had a spontaneous initiation of Kundalini awakening unrelated to activities. These transpersonal experiences and processes can start anywhere, anytime, if one is ripe, if one has reached that place in the soul's journey when profound awakening is called for.

The actions of Kundalini are often misunderstood, even by those steeped in yoga. Swami Muktananda, a Kundalini yoga master I studied under in the 1970s and early '80s, had a very powerful Kundalini awakening when he was thirty-nine. It happened after many years of yoga practices and intense austerities, when he met a master who could awaken Kundalini. Even with his extensive background in yoga and meditation, his initial experiences were so challenging to all his yogic attainments and beliefs that he literally ran away from his master, Swami Nityananda, thinking he had disgraced his yogic heritage! Because Kundalini and the spontaneous yoga that develops from its full awakening was misunderstood and rarely talked about back then, Swami Muktananda didn't have the understanding to properly see that what was happening to him was one of the most sought-after forms of initiation a yogi could ever hope to receive. It was in fact the culmination of his many, many years and lifetimes of dedicated practice.

Even now, when spontaneous awakenings appear to be more frequent, people who are uninformed about Kundalini may initially be fearful of this power. Accurate knowledge about the unfolding of this process can provide enormous comfort. It allows people to relax and receive the extraordinary gifts and benefits Kundalini provides. Challenges remain, but fear doesn't have to be one of them.

Fear is why even Swami Muktananda had such a strong initial reaction, making him question his path. Fortunately Muktananda ended up retreating to a small meditation hut in a mango grove far away from people, and there he found an esoteric yogic text on Kundalini, left by a *sadhu* (a wandering yogi) that explained the extraordinary auspiciousness of all that he was experiencing.

Having the right understanding allowed him to go through, even surrender to, Kundalini's radically transformative process despite the challenges it entailed.

Without a full and deep understanding of Kundalini, the ego mind, our ordinary consciousness, is prone to reacting with fear and anger. Kundalini awakening can feel unwanted, out of our control. The ego very much likes to think it is the one in charge, the only one home within us. Suddenly, with Kundalini awakening, the ego is confronted with a powerful presence that is ego-alien, not the ego mind at all. This scares the ego and can even feel "life-threatening," so our ego scrambles to pull out all of its control strategies. However, fear and anger always make the situation worse, amplifying what we are feeling and the reactivity in the mind-body system. Fear and anger trigger the autonomic nervous system and provoke a cascade of neurophysiological responses related to the fight-flight-freeze stress response, which even further intensifies fear and reactivity. Lower-brain centers then hijack the higher-brain centers, causing emotionally driven, irrational, and at times catastrophic thinking. All because the ego mind is afraid of what it doesn't understand and what isn't under its control.

However, despite whatever reaction we might be having, the presence that the ego mind is encountering is the true Self, the Divine within. Kundalini is the power of the Self to know the very highest wisdom, beyond the mind and words. We're so used to being identified with the little self, the ego mind, that we've become completely alienated from our own sublime Self. Kundalini rectifies this, clearing the dis-ease that comes from being split off from our true and highest nature. Right understanding is essential for skillfully proceeding on the path of *Kundalini sadhana,* the ancient a path of disciplined adherence to practices empowered by Kundalini. And cultivating that right understanding is part of its tradition.

WHY ARE YOU ALIVE?

Understanding the enormous power and intent of Kundalini requires grasping the vast context in which Kundalini's boundless power of transformation and revelation operates. To get at this context, we need to step back and take a look at the fundamental question, What is the meaning and purpose of human life, of your life? Pursuing that question engenders a quest for knowledge, for deep wisdom — not simple facts or scientific theory. The quest for understanding the deepest meaning and highest purpose of human life has motivated seekers, philosophers, sages, and saints for all of history. Consciously engaging in your quest marshals energies and archetypal forces, enthusiasm and excitement, in support of your journey, perhaps your loftiest endeavor. An enormous treasury of wisdom illuminating answers to this fundamental question exists to support you. Humanity encodes deep collective wisdom in our myths and symbols, throughout all traditions and parts of the world. The mythic journey of the hero or heroine remains a powerful source of such wisdom and deep understanding.

To make the profound nature of your path through life come alive in this moment, look at your life as a grand mythic journey, your own epic tale of *your* quest. Of course you'll have to consider carefully where you are going and what you are searching for on your journey. Who are you really? Why were you born? Where are you going? What are you searching for? What is the meaning of your life? If you take a few moments to carefully think about these questions, you've very simply opened your mind to discovering profound insights about your life. Staying with those questions, really pondering them, thrusts us forward on a journey of discovery. This is your quest, your great personal mythic journey. To succeed, to discover and fully live the realization of the greatest meaning and purpose of your life, you must consciously choose complete engagement with your quest. Many times along the way, you will find yourself questioning what you've considered to be true, or were told was true, in order to discover what really is true. There will be challenges along the way. No great quest is without danger or without the demand for sacrifice. Sacrifice makes life sacred, an ancient truth too often neglected in this age.

Joseph Campbell wrote in his brilliant work on the archetypal quest, *The Hero with a Thousand Faces:*

It has always been the prime function of mythology and rite to supply
the symbols that carry the human spirit forward, in counteraction
to those other constant human fantasies that tend to tie it back. In
fact, it may well be that the very high incidence of neuroticism among
ourselves follows from the decline among us of such effective spiritual
aid. We remain fixated to the unexorcised images of our infancy, and
hence disinclined to the necessary passages of our adulthood.[2]

You will be amazed by the wisdom that comes from within as you note your reflections on these questions. You might even want to begin a journal where you record the answers that come to you. Perhaps without knowing it, by simply asking the questions, you've engaged the archetypal powers of wisdom known by various names in different traditions—Sophia, Saraswati, Jnana Shakti, bodhicitta—and invited Kundalini to begin illuminating the deep mysteries of your life. It is within the context of answering the questions of what is the meaning and purpose of life, what is our true nature, what is the nature of the world and the Divine that Kundalini can best be understood. She is the innate power of Universal Consciousness that reveals the answers by giving us the direct experience of the highest states of consciousness possible, with all the wisdom that is found there.

INITIAL ENCOUNTERS

Many years ago when I started contemplating my quest and wondering when it started, I realized it began when I was a small child. My first encounter with what I now know as the Divine Feminine or the Feminine Face of God happened when I was very young and totally unaware of the meaning of the event. I was about three and a half years old, sleeping in my bed, and a booming thunderstorm awakened me in the middle of the night. I loved thunderstorms, as they were so alive, powerful, and unpredictable. I felt excited by the flashes of lightning and the pounding thunder. In the background, I could hear my older brother and sister sleeping soundly in our shared bedroom.

As I opened my eyes in the darkened room, I saw a beautiful woman standing beside my bed looking over me. Her form illuminated itself against the night as though she were comprised solely of light. Her face was strikingly sweet and loving as she looked over me with great tenderness. I thought this must be my mom. No one else ever looked at me like that and made me feel so secure. I just looked at her for a while. She didn't say anything. She simply stood by me as the thunderstorm boomed on. I noticed that as the room lit up with the lightning flashes, she would flicker and fade. When her light mixed with the lightning, she could hardly be seen. It was only in the dark that she was clearly visible. That was very unlike Mom! Was this really Mom?

In a little voice I said, "Ma?"

She didn't respond; she just kept smiling benevolently at me.

"Ma?" I said a bit louder. Still nothing. Beginning to panic I yelled, "Mommy!"

I heard my parents' bedroom door open across the hall. The "Lady of Light" stood there looking at me as I heard my mother's footsteps coming toward my room. The instant my mother entered our bedroom, the radiant figure vanished. Mom said it was nothing but a dream. But I knew better. For years I talked to my mother about the "Lady of Light," as I called her, who visited me during the thunderstorm. I didn't know then that I would see her again many years later.

Growing up on Long Island, New York, I was very successful in school. I worked a full-time job in addition to devoting myself to my studies in order to save for college. The prevailing motivators for people I was growing up with—facing competition, proving yourself, and striving for material gain—didn't speak to the needs of my soul for leading a meaningful life.

When I was eleven or twelve, I had another mysterious experience. I was up on the roof of our house, one of my favorite places, lying on my back, lost in the spaciousness of the sky, the clouds drifting by, the intense blue that outlined their brilliant white, when suddenly a voice from within told me I would die when I was twenty-four. It said I wouldn't live to see my twenty-fifth birthday. The voice was matter-of-fact, without emotion, and in my state of reverie I wasn't trouble by it. Twenty-four seemed nearly middle-aged to me at the time, and with all the threats of nuclear war that had people building fallout shelters, who knew if I would live that long. So I just continued to watch the clouds, enjoying the feeling of being as expansive as the sky.

At the end of high school, I was awarded a full academic scholarship to a state university, but as I left for college, all the big questions remained as I longed for meaning in my life: Who am I, why was I born, and what is the meaning of life?

In my first year of college, I began to delve into yoga and meditation. Within two months of beginning daily yoga practices during the summer before my second year of college, I was feeling better than I had in years. The counter-culture lifestyle I had been living, typical of the late 1960s, had already negatively impacted my body. Yoga was putting it back into shape. Meditation detached me from the tyranny of my mind and its self-defeating patterns, while giving me ways to use it more successfully. I was meeting people for whom the Divine was alive and directly experienced. They didn't call it the Divine or God; rather, using the Eastern traditions' terminology, they called it Universal

Consciousness—omniscient, omnipotent, all-embracing Consciousness. It wasn't hard to recognize this was God; God without distracting names or forms. I really felt blessed to have found the approach the Eastern traditions offered. It reinvigorated me, and I began to look forward to beginning anew as a sophomore. Then just weeks before the start of the academic year, an amazing event occurred.

I was living with my parents at the time in their new house in rural Connecticut, far away from where I grew up on Long Island. I used to go to bed early in order to get up at 5 a.m. for yoga and meditation. In the middle of the night, I awoke for no apparent reason, and as I opened my eyes and looked past the foot of the bed, I saw standing in the doorway my Lady of Light! She stood there just as she had sixteen years earlier in our other home. Her radiance was exquisite. I was completely captivated by her as I stared at her countenance. Gentle, soft light emanated from her every feature and from her diaphanous, flowing robes. Tender love, all-enveloping, profoundly caring love—beyond measure—poured from her and wrapped around me like a warm blanket. Tears ran down my cheeks. I felt like she had been there guiding me, protecting me, and enabling me to survive the struggles my life had included up to that point.

Now that I had chosen to engage consciously in my quest through yoga, this was her time to reveal herself to me once again. I took it as an incredibly auspicious sign, assuring me I was headed in the right direction. I couldn't keep my eyes off her as I lay in my bed, breathing deeply, almost as if I was trying to inhale her. I didn't want to speak and risk losing her. After ten or fifteen minutes, finally I spoke aloud, "I know you, I remember you." She continued to stand there, showering me with her radiant presence. An indescribable joy welled up inside me as tears continued to stream down my cheeks. No more words were necessary.

Eventually I closed my eyes, sinking into meditation, dissolving into light, and then into a state beyond the mind. I rested in a comfort I had never experienced before. It came with the security of knowing I was protected and guided in a most miraculous way. Years would pass before I learned that we all have the same guidance and protection available to us. Fortunately, I wouldn't have to wait another sixteen years before experiencing her presence again.

I began pursuing yoga and meditation with more and more discipline and dedication. My practice honed my body and mind to such an extent that I maintained straight A's even while going to school full time, working full time, and doing volunteer work. I graduated magna cum laude from the University of Connecticut. My yoga and meditation practices continued. During those years, I studied under a few of the contemporary Eastern gurus on the scene at the time. Usually after following their practices for a year or two, my practice would plateau or in some way the teacher would betray their own teachings and show they didn't have the self-mastery they professed to have.

By 1975, I was feeling discouraged by the lack of leadership available to me and feeling very stuck without it. I was reading Saint John of the Cross, the great Christian mystic, and his words about the necessity of having a teacher concerned me. He said a soul "on its own without a master is like a burning coal which is left to itself; it loses its glow and grows cold."[3] I was in danger. I needed the fire only a real master could bring, but so far all I had found were tragically flawed teachers. The *dharma* (the right action) of a true teacher is selfless service. There's a humility that goes with that. When I'd see arrogance, capriciousness, power games, sexual misconduct, or substance abuse dressed up in the emperor's new clothes of the teacher's perfection, I'd leave. My own naiveté and projections would play into this dynamic as well. I wanted someone who could hold the projection of my highest Self, my Buddha nature, and show me how to take that projection back inside, not take advantage of it for their own self-inflation. There are true masters who can carry that projection in a selfless way, and they always turn the seeker back to the source within.

Eventually, I met someone who told me about an extraordinary master of meditation, a *swami* (monk) from India. He was reputed to be able to awaken Kundalini, a very rare ability even among accomplished yogis, though at the time I really didn't know what that meant. In the late summer of 1976, I met Swami Muktananda at an ashram in upstate New York where he was giving programs. My meeting with him wasn't any different from that of tens of thousands of people who had met him during his previous world tours or would meet him in his subsequent world tours. Like many people who came to Swami Muktananda, I had no idea of the enormity of the moment or what was to unfold from that almost casual happenstance.

After the program, a long greeting line formed with everyone who wanted to meet him or receive his blessings. I joined the *darshan line,* as it is called in Hindu culture (*darshan* means "to see"). When I stood before him, I could hardly make sense of what was occurring inside me. My mind was saying, "Oh well, here's another guru, another swami. I've met them before. I doubt anything will be different." Simultaneously, my heart and body were trembling with excitement. My heart was saying, "This is it! Somehow he's got it!" without really knowing what *it* was! His eyes were unlike any eyes I had ever looked into—all at once they were jovial and compassionate—completely unfathomable. He used the brush of a wand of peacock feathers to greet and bless people, which was strangely energizing and quieting at the same time. After feeling the brush against my body, he gave me the mantra that everyone received for meditation: Om Namah Shivaya (I bow to the Divine within). I walked away feeling so light that it was as if I was several feet off the ground. I couldn't figure out what happened. I left him to return home, not knowing that this marked the awakening of Kundalini in this life for me.

The next day Swami Muktananda returned to India. Though I felt euphoric for several days, I put the whole event aside and went back to the Jungian analytic training and psychotherapy training I was pursuing along with my meditation and yoga practices.

AWAKENED KUNDALINI: YOUR INNER GUIDE

At that time I had no appreciation of what an extraordinary power Kundalini is or what gifts come through her awakening and unfolding. She is at the very heart of all forms of yoga. Shankaracharya, the eminent eighth-century sage of Advaita Vedanta (a non-dual school of Hindu philosophy[4]), wrote an ecstatic prayer, entitled *Saundaryalahari,* proclaiming the supreme power of Kundalini. In this text, he states that all knowledge, all wisdom, all inspiration, and all creativity—musical, poetic, literary, artistic, as well as union with the Divine—come through the power of Kundalini alone.[5] For this reason, the awakening of Kundalini is the esoteric goal of all forms of yoga; and the wise yogi yearns for the blessing of *shaktipat,* the term for the descent of grace that awakens Kundalini. Awakened Kundalini is the indispensable guide, the inner master guru, who brings the seeker to the highest state of attainment.

Kashmir Shaivism is another non-dualistic school of yoga and philosophy that developed in eighth-century India. Muktananda was one of the great teachers who spread the wisdom and powerful practices of Kashmir Shaivism in the West. It views the universe as pure Consciousness, or *Shakti,* taking on all shapes and forms by its own volition. Shakti is power, the energy of the universe that is also Consciousness itself. The Shaivite school presaged Einstein's discovery that all matter is in fact energy, bound energy, assuming the form of concrete matter. The enlightened sages knew this thousands of years before modern science.

The ancient Kashmir Shaivite text, the *Kularnava Tantra,* states that without shaktipat there is no liberation or Self-realization.[6] The descent of grace may happen spontaneously and unexpectedly or through the power of a master of genuine attainment, as happened to me when I met Muktananda. In some cases shaktipat is received through contact with a mystic guide who appears in one's dreams or meditation, as with the Lady of Light who appeared to me when I was young (numerous people have told me about their experiences of the Lady of Light as well!). Kundalini can also be awakened through a mantra or the practices learned from an accomplished spiritual teacher. It may even have been awakened in a past life and is continuing to unfold in this life. In short, no one person or practice is the sole available means of receiving the descent of grace, the awakening of Kundalini. The Divine is too generous to put such limitations on her accessibility.

The transmission of Kundalini through shaktipat is likened to what happens if you are lost in the dark and have only an unlit candle in your hand. If you are fortunate to encounter someone with a lit candle, they can pass their flame to your candle. Your candle is easily lit from the one that is already ablaze. Without the gift of that flame, you might have to labor for a very long time to find the means to manually light a fire to light your candle. Shaktipat ignites the fire of Consciousness within you that illumines your way back to the Self.

A couple of months after that brief encounter with Swami Muktananda in 1976, I entered the hospital for simple outpatient knee surgery. I was due out the same day, but a week later I was still in the hospital and the knee surgery hadn't been done. The routine screening x-ray for anesthesia that was done the morning I entered the hospital showed two fist-sized growths in my chest. Many tests and biopsies were done, and at first the doctors thought I might have lymphosarcoma. If I did, I was told it would be terminal. They speculated that I would likely be dead in two to three months, just before my twenty-fifth birthday. The memory of my twelve-year-old self, lying on the roof, and hearing a voice from within me speak of my death at the age of twenty-four, came rushing back. Only now twenty-four didn't sound very old! I was completely shocked when I heard the news and drew on my meditative and contemplative practices to try to make sense of what was unfolding. I watched as fear would arise and subside, along with sadness at not being able to complete this life in the way I had imagined, including leaving my fiancé before we even had a chance to get married. But I also felt such wonder about it all, the voice, where had that come from twelve years earlier, the Lady of Light, Muktananda—how did this all fit together?

I began thinking about my life and the lessons that were being presented to me. I was an avid backpacker and rock climber. These outdoor activities provided the metaphor for life as I saw it. You struggled up to the top of some mountain, enjoyed the view and the accomplishment, went downhill, and began looking for the next mountain. Self-effort and struggle dominated my perspective on life. I had learned to enjoy exerting myself in this way. But now I was encountering situations in which only a kind of surrender and letting go would work. They were very difficult for me despite my training and practice in psychology, yoga, and meditation. As I lay in my hospital bed one evening, I thought of the meditation master I had briefly encountered. People called him *Baba*, which simply means "father" and is routinely used in India when speaking to revered male elders. His image and presence felt so vivid, and I began a conversation with him in my mind. I was feeling so overwhelmed by this challenge of facing death, and I said, "Baba, I don't really know who you are. In fact, I don't think I know *what* you are, but I have no one else to turn to. I pray that you'll be able to help me. I don't have anything to offer you but this life of mine and even that may not amount to much. I gladly surrender it to you. Please show me a way through this."

Within a few moments my mind became very still, and I fell into a deep state of meditation. I felt I was in the radiant presence of both Baba and the Lady of Light. An orb of light surrounded them and me while all else disappeared. The profound serenity and the feeling of being watched over by them put all concerns about my future out of my mind. It felt as though a powerful energy was washing through my body, leaving it very relaxed and refreshed. I came out of the meditation hours later knowing everything would be fine, without knowing what "fine" would look like. I knew I would be at peace regardless of what happened. I offered a prayer of heartfelt gratitude to Baba and my Lady of Light before falling asleep in my hospital bed.

After several more days of testing and exploratory surgery, the doctors changed their diagnosis to a disease called *sarcoidosis,* not cancer, and as one doctor crassly said, "This one might not kill you until you're in your fifties!" Because of the transcendent light and grace I had experienced in that meditation while lying in my hospital bed, I knew I had nothing to worry about. Within a few months all traces of this disease disappeared too.

FOLLOWING KUNDALINI'S GUIDANCE

Kundalini awakening initiates the unique processes of purification, transformation, and revelation that only Kundalini can engender. Latent diseases can be brought up to be dispelled, as happened with me. Body karmas and relationship karmas are also old patterns of bound energy that may need to be released in order for you to experience the fullness of the Divine's creation and your Self as Creator. Those patterns that aren't dissolved or released are transformed by the wisdom, compassion, and love that Kundalini, your own sublime nature, embraces your life with. Because these patterns and karmas are unique for each individual, the details of the way in which Kundalini's processes of purification and transmutation unfold are also unique. You won't, nor do you need to, experience exactly what I or someone else experienced. Kundalini moves each seeker through the experiences that their karmas have shaped. All you need to do is learn to follow her lead. That is the essential task of Kundalini yoga born from awakened Kundalini. Meditation, other yoga practices, study, and contemplation, done with the guidance of a deeply practiced and selfless mentor, all work to refine the mind and your ability to discern the call of Kundalini arising within.

As a result of Kundalini awakening, I was having many powerful meditation experiences that further inspired me to look for a way to live a life dedicated to intense practice and service. During meditation and chanting the mantra Om Namah Shivaya, all sense of "me" would dissolve and merge my awareness in boundless fields of light suffused with ecstasy and all-embracing love. I would come back to ordinary consciousness, sometimes after hours, to find my body sitting in my meditation room, swaying back and forth, tears of unspeakable joy streaming down my face. My heart opened to such compassion and empathy for the suffering of others that it was unbearable not to be able to relieve people of it. I was living and working in a therapeutic community helping young adults with long-term mental illnesses and addictions. It was painfully clear how limited we are in relieving suffering. Yet Muktananda, like so many other great sages, saints, and seers, had dedicated his life to becoming free and in doing so was able to pass on a way for thousands and thousands of others to know that same blissful freedom.

A little more than a year after getting out of the hospital, I left my job, my fiancé, and everything else to fulfill my inner promise to offer my life in service to God through serving Muktananda. I had never told him anything about what had happened. In fact, my only contact with him had been that brief moment on the greeting line eighteen months earlier. It was difficult for me to leave everyone and everything I loved, but my soul demanded it of me. I told family and friends I was going to India to become a monk. My fiancé did her best to understand, but couldn't escape the pain of me leaving her.

I made it to Swami Muktananda's ashram in rural India, thoroughly exhausted from a thirty-six-hour flight, eleven-hour jetlag, and the attendant ordeals of traveling for hours through the Indian countryside in a three-wheel motor scooter. In my bedraggled state, I was immediately brought to Baba. I told him I had left everyone and everything because I felt that in order to really give myself to God and to live a life of the spirit, I had to renounce everything, become a monk, and spend the rest of my life in service. I was terribly serious. Fortunately Baba wasn't. He was humorously serious. Baba looked at me warmly and laughed. He said, "You can have them both, the worldly and the spiritual life." He paused and waited for that to sink in. The look on my face must have been something to behold; I felt like massive stone curtains were crumbling and falling away from my mind and vision.

Baba then said, "The worldly and the spiritual are not opposed; there is no reason to give up your life in that way." His words blew open my heart. I felt as if I might explode with joy. I left his presence with a lightness that nearly had me flying back home.

I was so excited by this turnaround that I felt I should leave immediately and return to my fiancé and career. I started packing again the next morning. Luckily, a friend brought me back to the ground and pointed out that since I had traveled halfway around the world to be with this great master it would be best if I stayed a few weeks to learn all that I could. There was no hurry; my boss, a Jungian analyst and mentor to me, had said I could have my job back if it became apparent that monkhood wasn't my path. The rigorous ashram schedule supports everyone's intention to be completely absorbed in sadhana, deepening their knowledge and direct experiences while eradicating the bonds of ego through seva, selfless service.

I would get up at 3:30 a.m. for meditation. Then at 5:00 a.m., I would go to the temple with hundreds of devotees to do morning *arati*, ritual devotional practices which included honoring the Divine through a ceremony of waving *arati* lights, lit ghee lamps, symbolizing the divine light of individual and Universal Consciousness, and chanting a half-hour Sanskrit hymn. It is among the most moving and inspiring practices I've ever done. Even after having done it literally thousands of times by now, I still can be overcome by tears of love, so powerful is this ancient practice for invoking Shakti.

I was new to the practice back then and was overwhelmed by the love and devotion that would arise. Nothing in my Western practices of religion or meditation compared with it. I was also deeply moved to see that men could be openly devotional and expressive of love and joy in relation to the Divine. My heart and soul expanded and sang on so many levels! After about three weeks in the ashram, it was time for me to go back, with Baba's blessings, and bring home the riches of the practices and teachings I had received from him.

When I arrived back in the States, I returned to my previous position as a therapist and program director at a Jungian psychiatric treatment center. Fortunately, my fiancé also welcomed me back! She knew I always loved her and only left because I was struggling to discern how to follow Kundalini's lead, how to live a life totally dedicated to sadhana and selfless service. Muktananda was guiding me to develop the discrimination and self-discipline necessary to do this. A few months later I married her. Over time Muktananda helped me to see that the outer obstacles I wanted to remove from my life through the renunciation involved in becoming a swami were actually the very aids I needed in this life to fully experience God and to learn to serve as an instrument of God's love.

During the next several years I watched with amazement as the transformative process of meditation unfolded in my life by Kundalini's grace. The changes I experienced and the ones I saw in countless others who had experienced Kundalini awakening led me to do my doctoral research on the dimensions of psychological change and spiritual growth that people experienced through their practice of a Kundalini-based yoga.[7] The research study was the culmination of my PhD studies in the clinical psychology track of the Department of Psychoeducational Processes at Temple University, where I was awarded a fellowship to study as a University Scholar.

In the spring of 1986, I was working on my dissertation and faced the task of writing about Kundalini as a part of my thesis. Suddenly, I confronted the fact that I really knew very little about Kundalini. Despite practicing a yoga based on the awakened Kundalini for a decade, despite experiencing profound states of meditation, despite hearing numerous lectures on Kundalini, reading countless books, and even lecturing on Kundalini myself, I couldn't say that I truly, fully understood Her or knew how this Divine power worked. For the most part, I simply felt awed by the transformations wrought by Her in myself and others. I was very familiar with the term Kundalini and concepts related to it, but that's no substitute for deep and complete knowing. By naming phenomena and accepting an authority's (scientific, religious, or yogic) explanation of them, we demystify them, even if they really are still a mystery. Kundalini had become familiar, but as I approached the task of writing about Her, I was once again humbly aware of what a mysterious power She truly is.

C. G. Jung wrote, "When you succeed in the awakening of Kundalini, so that she starts to move out of her mere potentiality, you necessarily start a world which is totally different from our world: it is a world of eternity."[8] It is into that archetypal world that our quest leads us. To understand the profound nature of the archetypal power of Kundalini, it is important to consider how the Divine Feminine, the Great Goddess, has been understood and related to in human history. That is the context within which we encounter Her.

THE GUIDANCE OFFERED IN *AWAKENING KUNDALINI*

This book is focused on helping your ordinary mind, with its constructed sense of self, begin to unfold, or further unfold, the power of Kundalini within you. This book is also a tool to help you appreciate the magnificent workings of Kundalini: how She creates and sustains the universe, how She creates bondage and dissolves it in radical freedom, awakening us to our unbroken unity with all beings and all creation. Kundalini accomplishes all this while transforming the mind-body into a selfless servant of the Divine. By better understanding Kundalini, we discover that it is in our best interest to learn how to follow her lead and surrender to her wisdom.

People new to Kundalini will find maps for getting oriented to her domain and instructions on some of the trails to follow and some to avoid. People already experienced in the ways of Kundalini may find valuable insights and ways of communicating about Kundalini that help others appreciate what you are experiencing. The focus of this book is on understanding the breadth and depth of Kundalini's dynamic processes and on developing practical, grounded ways of cultivating the disciplines of body and mind necessary to strengthen the channels for the potent energies released by Kundalini to flow through.

To support the mind's deepening understanding of Kundalini, we will look at the variety of ways in which She awakens and many of the characteristic types of experiences that people go through both in the awakening and unfolding phases of Kundalini's movements. We'll also look at the kinds of practices and attitudes we can cultivate to allow the transformative processes of Kundalini awakening to unfold as gracefully as possible. That doesn't mean this process will be entirely pleasurable for every individual. Transformation can at times be a turbulent process. Growth isn't always gentle and easy. We'll look at why that is and what can be done to ameliorate the difficulties.

This book isn't a substitute for working with an awakened and skillful teacher, but because many people are having Kundalini-type experiences, some subtle and some profoundly apparent, this book is here to give supportive guidance. *Awakening Kundalini* isn't intended to be a scholarly tome with countless references and endnotes. I've provided a bibliography at the back of the book that includes additional resources to pursue. There is so much to learn about Kundalini—much more than can possibly be covered in one book. The seven-and-half-hour audio program that inspired this book, *Awakening Kundalini: The Path to Radical Freedom,* offers additional instructions and guided practices for awakening and integrating the potent energies that lie within you.[9]

In this book I'll take a panoramic view of Kundalini and her domain before getting into more of the details of how She manifests in our lives. In chapter 1, I'll expand the context for understanding Kundalini by viewing her connection to the Great Goddess and to archetypes of the Divine Feminine. If you look back in history, you can see that it was largely the Divine Feminine that formed humanity's earliest experience of the Divine. Evidence from ritual artifacts going back thirty thousand years demonstrate this.

Much of the yogic view of Kundalini focuses on the *inner* domain of consciousness and energy. In chapters 2 through 4, I'll explore this vast inner domain and journey of awakening that Kundalini traverses, which can be likened to the archetypal journey of the hero or heroine. The awakening of Kundalini, which I'll discuss further in chapter 5, is the awakening of your power of consciousness to go beyond the confines of the ego mind. This awakening transforms the ego, the mind, the body, and every other aspect of our lives. I'll bring in Western psychology and Jung's depth psychology, both of which offer valuable insights on the dynamics of what happens when the ordinary bound mind encounters archetypal, symbolic, transpersonal, and spiritual material.

Awakening our great innate consciousness happens in response to our soul's yearning for freedom from suffering and for knowledge of the deep meaning and purpose of life. It is through connecting to this longing that we can better understand and work toward this process. In chapter 6, I'll discuss these yearnings in the context of Kundalini awakening.

In chapter 7, I will offer a new perspective for understanding our awakening and growth by comparing and contrasting Western psychology with yoga psychology. Our understanding of what motivates us to do what we do and what shapes our thoughts and actions is deeply influenced by Western psychology. Yet yoga psychology differs from Western psychology in a number of important aspects for understanding Kundalini and how the awakening of this power impacts the mind and body and what drives us.

On the path of spiritual practice and working with Kundalini, the development of discrimination or discernment is critical. If you want to follow the highest, how do you discriminate between the promptings of Kundalini Shakti as the voice of your highest Self and your ego mind? Chapter 8 will explore how to develop that discrimination and the impact it has on virtually every aspect of spiritual practice and life. Then, in chapter 9, this understanding of how to exercise discernment will be explored through practices you can do along your path. These practices work with the ego mind and prepare the mind and body for Kundalini awakening, as well as for the deepening of Kundalini transformation once She has stirred from her slumber.

The Classical yoga of Patanjali, as discussed in chapter 10, supports our integration of practices that unfold the sublime power of Kundalini. The eight limbs of yoga embrace all of life and Kundalini empowers yoga practices in unimaginable ways. In this chapter, I'll discuss how all eight limbs, not just *asanas* (the yoga postures that many people are familiar with) are important components of Kundalini sadhana and give a template for an integrated spiritual life.

In chapter 11, I'll delve into meditation. The practice of meditation is central to both preparing for Kundalini awakening as well as for unfolding Kundalini's transformative processes. Your meditation practice doesn't have to be a traditional sitting meditation; there are many ways of becoming absorbed in the flow of Kundalini's energy.

Whether you want to learn to play an instrument, speak a new language, master a skill or body of knowledge, it is typically necessary to have a teacher who offers more than a book or manual ever could. In chapter 12, I'll look at the special role that the teacher plays in supporting you on the path of Kundalini's unfolding and how you might go about finding the right person to study with.

In chapter 13, I'll take a larger view of all the different types of practices recommended for working with Kundalini and how they fall into one of three categories for shifting consciousness out of bound states. These categories come from the wisdom of the Kashmir Shaivite tradition. This chapter will help you understand and choose the right practice for the right time.

Chapter 14 discusses the actions of Kundalini herself, the movements known as kriyas, which are part of the unfolding of Kundalini's transformative processes. Understanding these and skillfully coming into congruence with them is critical for the graceful unfolding of Kundalini.

Everyone's path includes confronting challenges and trials. In chapter 15, we'll look at the typical challenges the ego mind and life can bring us and how to become more skillful at working with them using sadhana practices. One of those challenges is the "shadow side" of the mind, the dark unconscious aspects of the mind that can blindside us. Fortunately the shadow also has its own light and jewels buried within it, which Kundalini takes special delight in uncovering. Illuminating and transforming our shadow is a very important process, which we will examine in chapter 16.

I've included a list of resources at the end of this book. Every one of the topics discussed in this book would require volumes of texts to fully study it. The recommended readings will provide you a means for expanding your knowledge at your own pace and guided by your own interests.

In writing about Kundalini, I'll also draw on my personal experiences of Kundalini awakening and unfolding, and my studies with masters from yogic, Buddhist, Jungian, and shamanic traditions, as well as what I've learned from the many people who have sought me out to support them in their Kundalini processes. They have given me the privilege of seeing the deep workings of Kundalini's grace and revelation in manifold ways.

I refer to Kundalini as "She" or as "Her" for two reasons: In the yogic tradition this power is known as the feminine face of the Divine, a form of the Great Goddess. Secondly, like countless other seekers, I've been given direct experiences of her Divine Feminine forms, including her living presence, which is right here, right now.

Having an interest in Kundalini, seeking to learn more about Kundalini, and seeking to experience for yourself her immense power are already signs of her grace calling you home to your divine nature. May this book and all you encounter through it serve to bring you closer to radical freedom, to the boundlessly loving, compassionate, joyous and creative state of who you truly are.

1

Kundalini and the Great Goddess

Kundalini Shakti is one of the feminine faces of the Divine. In other words, Kundalini is an archetypal form of the Goddess. The Goddess, also known as the Great Mother, has been worshipped for over thirty thousand years, and symbolic representations of Kundalini go back thousands of years. Kundalini is seen as feminine, but not simply female in the sense of gender; She's seen as the archetypal form of the Divine Feminine because of the functions, powers, and processes associated with Kundalini. Kundalini Shakti is that which gives birth to everything, sustains and nurtures all creation, and welcomes it all back into herself as these ephemeral forms dissolve into Her once again. This Power of Consciousness known as the great goddess Shakti Kundalini, also known as Mahakali, Maha Kundalini, and many other names, is that which gives birth to all forms out of herself. She also gives birth to the forms of consciousness, forms of limited being, in order to know what it is to inhabit those bound forms. She has the unlimited Consciousness to transcend and embrace them, to know limitations *and* to know Infinite Being. These words attempt to point to an unimaginable state, a state that the ordinary mind, as one of those bound forms, will never know.

Shiva, the "auspicious one," is the transcendent, Infinite Consciousness that is inseparable from Shakti. In the system of Shaivism, He is the male counterpart to Shakti, God inseparable from Goddess. Shiva is the eternal, formless, transcendent, and ever-blissful One. His power to create, sustain, dissolve, conceal, and reveal is Shakti, the eternal power of Consciousness, always united with the transcendent formless One, Shiva. He is Shakti's formless dimension. She is his all-knowing creative power. The great sage of Advaita Vedanta, Shankaracharya, begins his hymn of praise to Shakti Kundalini, the Saundaryalahari, by proclaiming that the Auspicious One, Shiva, is incapable of creating or even moving without Shakti.[1] Shiva and Shakti are the universe of formlessness and form. There is nothing outside of them, separate from them. They allow only themselves into their transcendent domain. Thus to know the highest, one must completely dissolve back into the Source.

Shakti will take on any number of forms to usher seekers through her gate from the finite to the Infinite. She can become the masculine form of gods, feminine forms of goddesses, forms of mantras, yantras, guardians, paths, traditions, and more. All forms issue from Her. Some people wonder why, with their Kundalini awakening, they primarily have visions of Shiva or Krishna, Hanuman or Ram, Buddha or Jesus, or other male forms of the Divine, or why they don't perceive forms at all, but rather clouds of Light suffused with Loving Consciousness. The list of Shakti's possible creations is endless! She will appear in ways that will help the seeker move forward. It's important to let go of any preconceptions of how the Goddess should appear, let go of how we would like Her to appear, and receive Her as She chooses to appear, even if in the moment that is simply as a thought. Everything arising in the mind, including the mind itself, is Shakti.

FORMS OF THE GODDESS

The Goddess comes to seekers in many forms. As Kundalini, She is the power that brings the highest attainment—and She appears in the Hindu tradition as Shakti. But She goes by many other names. In the Buddhist tradition, we also see the Goddess revered as the source of all Buddhas. The Heart Sutra, one of the foundational scriptures of the Buddhist tradition, is called the Bhagavati Prajnaparamita Hridaya—*Bhagavati* means "the Great Goddess." It is the Great Goddess's highest wisdom, the heart-essence of wisdom that is referred to in the Heart Sutra. It's seen as the great mother who produces all *tathagatas,* "all those that go beyond," in other words all Buddhas and all their wisdom. Seeing emptiness in form and form in emptiness, Buddha's wisdom and attainments are born from Bhagavati, from the Great Mother. Thus, in the Buddhist tradition too, there's the recognition that the Divine Feminine is the one who gives birth to this wakefulness of Buddha mind, whether that awake one is in the transcendent domain or in the earthly domain as a walking Buddha.

In the West, one of the Goddess's forms is that of Wisdom. She is the Goddess Sophia and is revered for her great gifts of learning and spiritual insight. Philosophers—from the Greek *phileo Sophia,* which means "lovers of wisdom"—worship Her by pouring ablutions of attention on Her through contemplation and study.

The strong patriarchal religious traditions from the Middle East essentially banished the Goddess. The Divine Feminine appears in a reduced form as Mother Mary and through her icons of the black Madonnas—a fitting image for the Goddess having been pushed into the deep shadows.

The non-dual yogic traditions and Kashmir Shaivism recognize that all attainments come through the grace of Shakti Kundalini. All forms are her form because She is the Universal Creative Power, the one who creates all forms from herself; there is no "other." Thus all mystical traditions as forms of knowledge are her traditions; all wisdom is her wisdom and that universalist understanding is part of what unfolds with the awakening of Kundalini—these are her sublime gifts. That doesn't mean all wisdom is the same or that all traditions lead to the same attainment. Not every wellspring is pure, not every stream makes it to the sea. When you walk into a jewelry store, you see many forms of gold, but they are not all the same even if they are all gold. Looking closer you see some things are made of pure gold, some are alloys of lesser value. Through Kundalini's grace, She empowers one with the discrimination to see through the finite to the Infinite, to see through forms to the formless. More than that, She is calling you, begging you, to join Her in this sublime, ecstatic state of wakefulness!

THE GREAT GODDESS ACROSS TIME

Evidence that the Great Goddess has been known and revered goes back over thirty thousand years. For all but the last five to seven thousand years, She reigned supreme. Most of human history is in fact "Herstory." In her book, *The Chalice and the Blade,* Riane Eisler traces what has happened in the evolution of spirituality across thousands of years. She begins by going back to the time when the worship and the understanding of the Great Goddess dominated the human psyche and human tradition, more than five thousand years ago. It's from that time that you see all the iconic forms and statues, often thought of as primitive statues, of the Goddess. They're found throughout civilization—from ancient India to ancient Europe. Goddess-centered consciousness demonstrated the archetypal Divine Feminine consciousness that generates and knows the rhythms and mysteries of life, death, and rebirth.

The Goddess knows what it is to create forms and life within herself, holding and nurturing, actualizing the potential in the seed, in new life, and bringing it forth, nurturing it with the milk from her own body. The ways of the Goddess were reflected everywhere in nature, and humanity lived with reverence for Her and attempted to live in harmony with the wisdom She revealed. For thousands of years, society was based on cooperation, being neither matriarchal nor patriarchal. For thousands of years, there were no fortifications or evidence of war. However, over time, a new form of consciousness began to develop in what Eisler calls the *dominator mode*.

The dominator mode was associated with patriarchal forms of religion and approaches to the Divine, which continue to persist to this day. The dominator mode also coincides with a shift in human culture where fortifications, battles, and wars between groups developed. That's what Eisler is referring to in the title of her book. She writes about the difference between the chalice and the blade. The chalice is a symbol of the Divine Feminine, the consciousness that holds and contains, that nurtures, that actualizes, versus the blade that cuts and severs, that differentiates, penetrates, and dominates. From my perspective, both are part of the full expression of Consciousness and forms that Shakti creates to express the complete spectrum of Consciousness. The pendulum has swung to an extreme and now is moving back to a center that integrates both modes of consciousness.

Eisler explains that as the dominator mode developed, there was a shift in understanding that was expressed in changes in religious traditions as well as other cultural and political structures. It radically changed the approach to the Divine Feminine. As the patriarchal dominator mode of consciousness began to flower, the Divine Feminine became more and more suppressed, so much so that in time, in some Middle Eastern cultures, the Goddess became known as the "abomination."

Furthermore, priestesses of the Goddess traditions went from being the high priestesses, revered and loved for their wisdom (such as Goddess Sophia), to being suppressed and distrusted for their power. They were thought of as witches. Some were hunted down because they had powers that weren't under the control of whatever the dominant patriarchal religious tradition came to be.

There are some Eastern cultures where the denigration of the Divine Feminine didn't happen. To this day the Goddess, the Devi, in many forms, continues to be worshipped and honored in India and other Eastern nations. Her power, her glory, her role as the one that draws us into Unity Consciousness continues to be recognized.

The patriarchal dominator mode or perspective changed the interpretation of some of the ancient symbols of the Divine Feminine, for instance, the snake. The snake was an ancient symbol of the traditions that honored the Divine Feminine and the Goddess. You'll see Her in ancient forms of the uroboros, a symbol of a snake looking like it's chasing its tail or eating its tail. It is a symbol of the Divine Feminine's ability to give birth and to be reborn like the snake shedding its skin. She is forever recreating herself. The circular form of the symbol of the uroboros implies the never-ending nature of many cycles. This was part of the wisdom of the Divine Feminine, knowing the cycles of life, being informed by them, and living in harmony with them. Some of the mysteries of the Divine Feminine were understood to be impenetrable, and it was only by the grace of the Goddess that one could enter the mysteries, that darkness, and gain direct knowledge that the ordinary mind and ordinary words would never illuminate or touch. The Goddess gave the fruit from the tree of knowledge, and the dominator form of a male god didn't like that!

Goddess Kundalini, as a quintessential form of the Divine Feminine power of consciousness, has been touched by those dominator modes that influenced the development of yogic traditions. There have been approaches in the yogic traditions that try to dominate Kundalini, to forcefully push Kundalini to do this or do that by prescribing endless exercises of forced breathing and body postures that are meant to bind and force Kundalini to go in a direction that the yogi wants Her to go. Not surprisingly, these are also traditions that often say Kundalini is dangerous and must be controlled. These were also the kinds of descriptions that have been applied to the Divine Feminine by patriarchal dominator approaches. But this power of Consciousness is indomitable, it isn't going to be suppressed; it always has its ways of coming out.

The wise seek to approach Her through reverence, love, and devotion, and then they gain the good graces of this power. Devotees that approach Kundalini as the Great Goddess with their loving devotion have an entirely different experience. They gain her boons, her gifts of enlightenment, without having to fear what may be provoked by some forceful, domineering practice. That attitude is key to understanding how we receive the gifts that this extraordinary innate power of Consciousness has to offer. It doesn't mean that our experiences of our karmas going up in flames may not be intense. But there's no need to exacerbate things with a willful egotistical attitude.

We're living at a time of the return of the Goddess. We need her wisdom to inform and inspire humanity to live cooperatively again if life on this earth is going to survive. We need her clarity of vision, her deep compassion, and her unwavering patience to live in harmony with each other and the environment. We need the awakened state of selflessness that Kundalini Shakti bestows, empowering people to recreate society, social structures, businesses, and economic systems on a cooperative model instead of the dominator mode that breeds destruction and war. The more She awakens people, the more individuals there will be transforming the collective consciousness of families, groups, towns, businesses, and countries. We are her organs of perception and action. Empowered by Her, we can see clearly and act wisely.

KALI: THE DARK GODDESS, MOTHER OF THE UNIVERSE

Kundalini is one of the great archetypal forms of the magnificent Goddess Kali. Kali, the Great Mother Goddess of the Hindu tradition, is the Source, the One that gives birth to all. Known as a slayer of demons, She destroys the army of mind-born delusions symbolized by demons that separate us from the Divine as our own true Self. Into our bound, limited, and contracted ego identities, She may strike terror, at times appearing as a coal-black, sword-wielding, blood-smeared dancer of death and destruction. To our Divine Self, Shiva, She is our supremely beautiful Beloved, our dear spouse, performing a ballet of incomparable grace, overwhelming us with love.

Kali is Shakti, spouse of Shiva. Ma Kali's story is profoundly meaningful. (Referring to Her as Ma is a devotional expression that recognizes Her as the

Great Mother, She who gives birth to all and protects all.) Shakti took the form of Kali when a horrific demon named Raktabija ("blood seed") was threatening to destroy the world. The demon won a boon from Lord Brahma that made him invincible by turning every drop of blood he spilled into ten thousand Raktabijas as soon as the drop of blood hit the ground. Wounding him only produced countless more demons. The gods went to Shiva for help, but he was immersed in his transcendent state and unavailable! His inseparable consort Shakti, ultimate power of the universe, answered their pleas for help and took the form of Kali. Kali went after Raktabija and all his clones, cut off their heads, and drank their blood before it could touch the ground. She vanquished them all, but then continued dancing her mad dance of destruction, destroying the bound forms of many non-demons. The gods went to Shiva to get him to stop her dance. He lay down beneath her feet, absorbing the power of her pounding steps as though they were mere love taps. She dropped her Kali form and revealed her exquisite nature as Shakti, adored by Shiva.

The demon is the archetype of the shadow side of the mind. What it reveals is that just like the thoughts of the mind, Raktabija's lifeblood has the power to give birth to thousands more Raktabijas. In the same way, the mind's thoughts appear to sprout more and more thoughts as soon as they seem to land. Even if one cuts them off in meditation, more sprout. Quelling the mind, dispatching the demon, requires the power of Shakti Kundalini. In this great mythic tale, Kali comes in and cuts off the demon's head. She drank all its blood before it could hit the fertile ground of existence. In other words, Kali Kundalini takes the life energy out of all the thoughts, desires, and delusions that plague the seeker and prevent the seeker from knowing pure union. Kali, as She's cutting off the heads, is symbolically cutting through the mind, cutting all the thoughts that are going to give birth again and again to bondage and delusion. She absorbs them into herself; in other words, She frees the life-force, the Shakti, from those bound forms. All forms are her creation. She alone has the power to dissolve all forms, releasing the energy, her energy, from them.

Kali wears a garland of fifty skulls around her neck. Those fifty skulls actually represent the fifty letters of the Sanskrit alphabet—the sounds and forms that make up thought, that are the basis of all creation. She's the one who takes the life-force out of them so that we can be free of them, as well as the one who gave birth to them to begin with. Taking refuge in Kali is taking refuge in that innate power to cut off the heads of the very thought forms, attitudes, beliefs, and all the limiting structures of the mind that catch us in delusion. Once cleared, She brings us to union again with the Infinite—as Kali does with her spouse Shiva. Even a myth like this, which may seem so bizarre and gruesome to the ignorant, has profound meaning for our sadhana, revealing what is involved with our spiritual practice moment by moment.

When you are doing *japa,* the practice of mantra repetition, of Om Kali Ma, her mantra, you are bringing your awareness back to Kali over and over again. You can do this practice right now or the next time you sit for meditation. Close your eyes and dissolve every thought into Om Kali Ma, Om Kali Ma, Om Kali Ma. (We'll go further into mantra practices in chapters 9 and 11.)

Kali's story shows that this magnificent dynamic is going on with every repetition of Om Kali Ma. As the throb of mantra, She cuts off all the thoughts, all the deluded thinking, all the bound attitudes and feelings that may have occupied the mind. Holding the mind in the refuge of mantra means holding the mind in a sacred place that is free of all the thought forms that the mind might have created its own bondage with. Every repetition of mantra is a movement of Kali's sword clearing and opening that spaciousness of awareness, freeing our energy and consciousness so that we can experience the fullness of who and what we are in each moment.

The great goddess Kali can never be understood by the intellect. Her essential nature is beyond the mind. Don't be surprised if your rational mind rebels and wants to go no further! Poets and mystics advise us that in order to know Her we must plunge into her luscious, radiant blackness and dive through our fear of the unknown into her overwhelming mystery, allowing ourselves to dissolve in her velvety midnight embrace. By her grace, we may know the unutterable truth of her love, even as we are annihilated by her infinitude.

JAI KALI MA

What mind can possibly approach you,
Much less grasp you, my beloved Kali!
This ordinary mind longs for you to be simple,
predictable, easily appreciated, a sweet divinity,
a demure goddess, lovely to look at, engendering kindness.
Instead you parade forth in gruesome reality,

unabashed, you unleash your limitless creative power,
thrilling the mind and body with overwhelming sensual delights,
propelling the spirit into awe-inspiring transcendent domains and
crushing us all in your jaws of time, decay and suffering.

You gave birth to ignorance and her offspring,
"lacking this" and "wanting that," populate the universe.
Is there nothing you don't delight in creating?
How is this poor mind ever going to truly worship you?
I set out to circumambulate your divine form,
    to do puja to you,
But lifetimes of effort have left me gasping,
seeing your infinitude spread out in all directions,
my mind and heart quiver with fear and adoration,
longing for annihilation in you, my beloved.

You demand full and total sacrifice,
not flower garlands and coins tossed at a statue,
not merely lighting candles and prostrating piously,
not sitting still as a corpse lost in the illusion
    of inside and outside.
No, you delight in swallowing all sense of separation,
Offer me your individuality you say,
Offer up your ego mind,
Offer up the waking, dream and deep sleep states!

This yoga is only for the insane
drunk on the nectar of Divine Love.
If you drink from the Holy Grail
you will drown in the end.

KALIDAS[2]

To this day Kali is worshipped around the world. She continues to be a living archetypal form of the Great Goddess who initiates seekers into the highest wisdom. A woman who was a dedicated Zen practitioner asked me about what she thought was a bizarre recurrent experience: It would happen after sitting for hours, when finally her mind and sense of self would begin to dissolve. She would always see what she described as a luscious, irresistible, black portal, glistening, and inviting. To her, it looked almost like a Georgia O'Keeffe black iris painting. She would be drawn into the blackness of that portal and disappear, and her ordinary mind and ego sense would be completely erased. That too is Ma Kali, Kundalini Shakti, dissolving the mind in the Infinite. She doesn't care what path brings you to her portal. She delights in taking whatever form will draw the seeker into union.

2

The Universe Within

The yogic system of psychophysiology gives a fascinating description of what is called the subtle body. The subtle body is an energy body that interpenetrates our physical body. Though many readers may be familiar with the subtle body, I'll go into more details about the energetic system, the chakras and nadis, later in this chapter. What is important to note is that it is within the subtle body that the dormant form of the energy of Universal Consciousness, referred to as Kundalini, resides. Once activated from her primal resting place in the subtle body, at a location near the base of the spine (muladhara chakra), the awakened Kundalini begins her work of transforming and purifying the subtle body and the physical body. Kundalini awakening can also occur at the level of the heart (anahata chakra) or at the level of the space between and above the eyes, the "third eye" (ajna chakra). However or wherever Kundalini awakens, the ensuing experiences and shifts in consciousness constitute the seeker's unfolding spiritual journey directed by their innate power of transformation and revelation.

Kundalini creates the subtle body, which serves as the matrix for creating the gross physical body. In the yogic paradigm it is the subtle body that creates the physical body. Within the yogic framework, it is critical to have a basic understanding of the subtle body in order to understand yoga, meditation, mantra, Kundalini, Kundalini awakening, and the profound transformative process of Kundalini unfolding. Because the subtle body isn't physical, it can't be perceived by our ordinary senses, making it seem especially mysterious and wondrous. What is often described as one's "aura" is a "visible" manifestation of the subtle body, but only visible to those with the subtle sense to perceive it. Acupuncture is a widely accepted form of medical treatment that scientific research has shown to be effective for treating several disorders. It works on the energy flowing through the subtle body, which affects the health of the physical body. Due to the limitations of scientific research, the underlying subtle energies haven't been detected by the gross physical instruments of measurement used in research.

This body is subtle compared with the gross body, through which we experience very concretely all the physical sensations our sense organs make available to us. The subtle body is the "body" of our mind, thoughts, feelings, emotions, intuitions, and other less commonly identified forms of energy such as *prana,* which are familiar to yogis and many yoga students but not to the uninformed or uninitiated. Our mind is so conditioned to think concretely when it encounters the word *body* that it tries to conjure an image like the concrete image of the physical body. But here *body* refers to nonphysical energy, centers of consciousness called *chakras,* conduits for energy called *nadis,* and functions of the mind. It's hard for the ordinary mind to remember that there is nothing physical or material about the subtle body. The gross physical body is the material projection of the subtle body.

The energy that flows through the subtle body is called prana in the yogic system. Prana is produced by Kundalini and is the enlivening power of both the subtle and physical bodies. It is a contracted, bound form of one aspect of Kundalini's power to create. Prana is defined in yoga as the life-force and is intimately connected to the breath. Thus, the yogic practice of pranayama, the control or restraint of prana, which is one of the eight limbs of yoga, focuses on breath regulation as a central practice for working with prana. As I work with people using biofeedback and yogic breath work, they discover that their agitated mind states are accompanied by shallow and faster breathing. From a yogic perspective, we could say their prana is disturbed, dysregulated. Regulating the breath has a powerful effect on the mind and our state of awareness. Research shows that slowing and deepening the breath in ways that yogis have prescribed for thousands of years, making the breath longer, more diaphragmatic and evenly paced, helps to calm the mind and changes brainwave patterns into more alpha rhythms associated with calmer, more relaxed states. This simple practice lowers blood pressure and stress hormones, enhancing cardiovascular functioning along with many additional positive effects. The racing mind slows down along with the breath. Though our energetic body is a very subtle realm, it is very real to us, just as our thoughts, emotions, attitudes, beliefs, dreams, and aspirations are quite real to us.

Science as a materialist discipline isn't able to research the non-physical nature of the subtle body and its energies, yet we are familiar with it in many appreciable ways through our mind, which is one of the central aspects of the subtle body. Science deals with the gross physical realm and can only detect physical correlates to thoughts and feelings—correlates such as brainwave patterns, respiratory rates, or electrodermal responses. A researcher using the most refined instruments attached to your skull may be able to give you data about the neuromuscular activity occurring while you are immersed in an experience, but only you know that at that instant you are recalling a tender moment of being held in the arms of a loved one. That kind of memory is not at all "subtle" or mysterious, yet the rich content of it, the potent impact it has on you, goes far beyond the ability of the most sensitive scientific instruments to measure. However, you already possess the most subtle and powerful instrument capable of apprehending such memories, feelings, and subtle phenomenon: that instrument is consciousness itself. Your conscious attention is your power of apprehension. It can be greatly developed and refined through meditation and awakened Kundalini.

THE SUBTLE BODY AND STATES OF CONSCIOUSNESS

During ordinary waking state awareness, our consciousness is almost entirely identified with the physical body. The subtle body phenomena of consciousness is primarily conditioned by and limited to the physical body during the waking state. We're aware of various physical sensations, feelings, and thoughts about ourselves that are rooted in the gender of our body, the shape it is in, and the functions or roles it is performing in our family, groups, or society. We are conditioned to think of ourselves as man or woman, fat or thin, son or daughter, husband or wife, boss or employee. In fact, we are so conditioned to think this way that we don't even think of it as conditioned. But from the vantage point of our consciousness freed from such conditioning through meditation, yoga, and Kundalini's grace, we can see what yogis and meditation masters have seen for millennia—that consciousness becomes conditioned to identify with the mind, body, and the roles we play. Sadly, for most people this comprises all of what they will give their attention to for their entire lives. But there's infinitely more to who we are and what we have available to experience and learn from.

The subtle body is another realm entirely. We experience the subtle body most exclusively when we are in the dream state of consciousness and in some meditative states. In the dream state, we leave the physical realm. The laws of physics no longer apply; gone are the constraints of ordinary time and space. We experience consciousness relatively free of the fetters of the physical body, but consciousness is still bound in certain ways. We're still identified with a limited sense of self, the ego mind, and the thoughts, feelings, and reflections of our physical body identity. At the same time, we can move through time and space in ways the physical body never can. In our dreams we fly, move back to the past, ahead to the future, or to some alternate present.

Because we are so identified with the body and waking state consciousness, the subtle body and the subtle realms of dreams, thoughts, feelings, imagination, and intuition are often disorienting. These realms may seem alien, perhaps even incomprehensible, to our waking state sense of self. Usually our waking state "I," the ego mind, dismisses or devalues our dreams and other unusual subtle body experiences, but through meditation, we can enter and explore the subtle realms quite consciously. The great yogic sages have done this and reported on the subtle, non-physical "physiology" of the subtle body. The ancient Shiva Sutras say that yogic realizations are amazing. When people directly experience aspects of the subtle body, the causal body, and the infinitude of the One, the source of all phenomena, for themselves, they are indeed amazed! We can read about such realizations in the lives of saints and sages of all traditions, from modern and ancient times. What is particularly stunning is to see that by the power of awakened Kundalini, ordinary people in everyday life have direct experience of yogic realizations such as hearing mantras arising within themselves, seeing the ephemeral nature of mind and body while resting in union with the eternal One, and discovering the boundless love and compassion that forever stand present with us, inviting us to revel in them and pass them on to all forms of our Self. The ultimate yogic realizations unfold beyond words in pure Unity Consciousness.

Not everyone will or needs to explore the subtle body in detail in order to complete their journey to the Infinite, but the yogic insights into the functioning of the subtle body and how it affects our states of consciousness and bodily states of health and disease are very useful in the lifelong course of spiritual practice.

Kundalini Shakti can bring your awareness into the depths of the subtle body during meditation. At the root of every physical sense perception, there's an even more subtle essence of each sense—in hearing, sight, touch, smell, and taste. Shakti might give you powerful experiences of the scent of divine ambrosia transporting you into sublime realms while you are in meditation. You might hear exquisite sounds, indescribable, that lie at the root, the essence of what our hearing is. There are tastes that outshine any taste in the world. There are experiences of sensuality that open up in meditative practices that make the most beautiful physical experiences pale in comparison.

A few years ago, I was contacted by a woman in her eighties and she said, "I don't know what's going on. I've been a meditator for many years, but now I've started having all this energy moving through me in meditation. I have orgasm after orgasm happening quite spontaneously. But I'm eighty-six years old! What am I supposed to do?" This was the gift of the Shakti unfolding a sublime experience for her and inviting her to know that the body also participates in the ecstasy of Shakti. One doesn't need to *do anything. That's always the ego mind's response, searching for something to do* with a phenomenon or experience. All the ego needs to do is watch with reverence and wonder, to sit as a witness and appreciate Shakti's magnificent gifts.

AWARENESS EXERCISE

After reading this, close your eyes and explore the subtleties that your consciousness is capable of becoming aware of. Take your time. Just as when you come inside from a bright sunny day into a dimly lit room and it takes your eyes time to adjust to the subtler level of illumination, your mind needs time to adjust from the gross level of stimuli through the senses to the very subtle levels of perception needed to directly experience the subtle body.

With your eyes closed, bring your awareness to your breath and allow it to gently slow and deepen while your attention follows the rise and fall of your diaphragm and the sensation of the air moving in and out through your nose. Mind and body are free to let go of any other thoughts or distractions to simply rest on the flow of the breath. After a few minutes of settling and allowing your mind to regain some of its subtle faculties, turn your attention to sensing the awareness of your body.

Become aware of your whole body, from head to toe, fingertip to fingertip, front and back; awareness fills and surrounds your body like a cloud of awareness.

Notice how your physical body rests within this cloud of awareness.

Notice how the flow of your breath comes and goes like waves moving through this cloud of awareness, waves of energy, waves of light, waves of vibrations. Enjoy watching and exploring the subtle body of energy and awareness.

You may notice the energy forms of thoughts and feelings as they arise and subside in the subtle body and how you can choose the energies you want to remain and dissolve and release those that don't serve your true nature.

You may notice the energy beneath bodily sensations, the touch of your clothes or the movement of air on your face.

You might notice the energy of sound and what happens as your ears pick it up or your body vibrates with it.

Explore your body of energy and consciousness for as long as you like.

OVERVIEW OF SUBTLE BODY COMPONENTS

Now that we've discussed the foundational concepts needed to understand the subtle body and how very different it is from the physical body, we can look more closely at the components of the subtle body, remembering that they are made solely of nonphysical energy, the power of consciousness, Shakti. We have to leave behind the ordinary mind's concrete ways of thinking and imagining as we look at the "anatomy" of the subtle body. We don't have a language for these nonphysical components of the subtle body, and we have to rely on metaphor, symbols, and images from the physical world, even though these are not at all physical.

Just as our physical body has conduits for vital fluids and nerve impulses, the subtle body has "conduits" for the energy of consciousness. These conduits are called nadis, and they circulate the living conscious energy of prana throughout our bodies. In meditation, the nadis may appear to the meditator like the filaments of light in fiber optics or a laser light show. They are exquisite! This is one of the many hidden realities She may reveal.

Where several nadis join together, the conduit is larger, like a bigger fiber-optic cable. In our physical body, the main nerve conduit running from the brain down to the base of the spine is the spinal cord, a great bundle of nerve fibers that connects the highest centers in the brain to the entire body. In roughly the same location in the subtle body, there is the main conduit of pranic energy, called the *sushumna nadi,* running from an area at the center of the head down to near the base of the spine. I'll discuss the sushumna nadi and the chakras in more detail in chapter 4.

The sushumna nadi is not only the major channel for the creative energy of Consciousness, Kundalini, to flow through; it is also the repository for all the past impressions left by our actions, both mental and physical. The sushumna nadi contains the impressions, called samskaras, of all our many lifetimes. In this way, it is the storehouse of all our *karmas,* all the consequences of our past actions that we have yet to experience. We're all familiar with CDs or DVDs. On a CD, millions of impressions are stored. When the laser light of the CD player mechanism passes over the CD, it picks up the patterns and converts them into music, pictures, video, or whatever it is that is stored on it. The sushumna nadi stores the information from countless impressions, the samskaras, of all our actions in energetic form. When the light of our individual consciousness passes through them, it picks up those patterns and manifests them. In this way, patterns of thinking, feeling, acting, relating, and creating are built up over lifetimes and reproduced again and again. It is these samskaras, the patterns and consequences of our own past actions, that bind consciousness to the forms of identity that we normally experience as our sense of self, our limited I-consciousness, each and every day.

Becoming fully liberated, radically free, requires that we become free of our samskaras and the limited forms of self that create them. This is the work of the awakened Kundalini. She does this in two ways. First, Kundalini moves through the sushumna nadi and lesser nadis, "erasing" the impressions stored there and releasing the energy bound up in those impressions. This extraordinary purification process then releases us from the patterns in our lives created by those impressions. Some of these are karmic impressions from past lives that bind us in particular ways related to those karmas. These affect the health and state of our body, the kinds of relationships we engage in, our family members and patterns of relationships, our work, the culture we took birth in to live out such karmas, mental patterns, and the like. All of these samskaras form the landscape of our individual existence. For example, from a yogic perspective, believing that possessing something will add to or give us happiness or fulfillment is a samskara based on ignorance that has built up over lifetimes and has tremendous power to shape our thoughts and actions. "I really need a new phone!" How many times have you heard an adolescent say that or something similar? Each person can substitute their own cravings and desires that they feel they so badly need, but the basic pattern of craving possessions, relationships, power, and so on is a deep samskara that meditation, yoga, and Kundalini awakening illumine and, over time, dissolve. Kundalini sets us free from the compulsive actions that drive the conditioned mind and that are so evident in our everyday lives and surrounding culture.

Secondly, Kundalini opens up states of consciousness to give us access to unbounded awareness, awareness of the transcendent Self, what some call God-consciousness or Buddha-mind. These are the altered states of consciousness, the experiences of mystical union and profound meditation that allow us to perceive that we are infinitely more than we think we are. They lead to the proclamation of the ancient Vedas: "I am Brahman," "I am the Absolute," or "Tat Twam Asi," meaning "Thou Art That," or the words of the Christian mystic, Saint Catherine of Genoa, "My Me is God, nor do I recognize any other Me except my God himself."[1] In order for that state of Unity Consciousness to become stable and fully manifest in our mind, body, and actions, the sushumna nadi and all the lesser nadis must be purified, cleansed of impressions and blocks that restrict consciousness to the confines of ordinary human experience. This is accomplished both by the actions of awakened Kundalini as well as by engaging in the disciplines and practices of your spiritual path.

3

Encountering Kundalini

Through the Heart, Beyond the Mind

ntellectual knowledge is not enough to really know Kundalini and her ways. The Eastern traditions emphasize the absolute necessity of direct experience. It's not sufficient to study yogic texts or to know that someone else at some time experienced the truth of yogic realizations. One has to experience it for oneself.

As I mentioned in the introduction, I felt I couldn't write anything about Kundalini for my doctoral research without that deeper knowing. I wanted to do the inner research and gain true knowledge. I needed to turn directly to Kundalini for the understanding for which I longed. I began to contemplate how best to approach Her. How could I open myself to receiving whatever wisdom She might share with me? I knew She was a part of me, but I was uncertain about how to invoke that part, how to relate to Her, how to directly connect with Her. I proceeded by going into meditation and contemplating these questions, trusting that She would bring to consciousness what I needed to know in order to move ahead. What came to mind were two related events from years earlier that made it clear how I should approach the goddess Kundalini.

In 1981, I heard a story about a renowned author on the topic of Kundalini who went to meet Swami Muktananda (who, as I mentioned, was known in part for his exalted visions of Kundalini and his devotion to Her). I was living in Muktananda's ashram in upstate New York at the time of this author's visit. The author too had visions of Kundalini, but to him She appeared quite unimpressive, looking like an ordinary woman, not like a goddess at all. As he waited outside the room where Baba was receiving visitors, he was totally astonished to have a vision of the goddess Kundalini entering the room where Muktananda was. Only this time She appeared in her most regal and resplendent form, magnificent and awe inspiring. The author was shocked. When he finally went in to speak with Baba, he asked why it was that She appeared so ordinary to him, while for Baba She came as the Goddess of the Universe. Baba replied simply, "Because I worship Her."

After I first heard that story I began contemplating what it means for an accomplished yogi to worship Kundalini. I kept wondering *how* a yogic master worshipped Kundalini. And why should a yogi want to? After a year, my mind finally gave up its vain attempts at piercing the mystery on its own, and I prayed to the inner guru, Shakti Kundalini, for an answer (Kundalini is the underlying power of the guru and functions from within each person as the inner guru). In a profound series of meditations, Kundalini, the great power of transcendent consciousness, showed me how worship (i.e., actively honoring and revering the divine power of grace) is the key to receiving all the wisdom She wishes to impart. This is the path of *bhakti yoga,* the yoga of devotion, where the worshipper and the worshipped merge, where duality surrenders through love to non-duality. On this path, the seeker and the Sought, lover and Divine Beloved, delight in the play of shifting back and forth between the sublime joy of dualistic worship and the ecstatic consummation of the worship in union.

The experiences that unfolded across two days and many hours of meditation revealed that the approach of loving devotion and worship of Kundalini invokes her boundless generosity and grace. For a yogi, true worship is to merge with the one you worship, whether that one is Shiva, Shakti, Tara, or any other face of the Divine. It is through worship and prayer, not reading and study, that Kundalini reveals the mysteries of the universe to the self-disciplined seeker. In answer to my prayer, She appeared as a series of six goddesses. I later learned that these were the goddesses of the six chakras that Kundalini manifests and moves through before returning to her primal form as the Maha Shakti, the great power, that takes the form of Mahakali, spouse of Shiva in the *sahasrara* (crown chakra). It is this highest power that dissolves the universe as

She merges into the Infinite and then creates it once again as She descends from that transcendent realm. Kali was the last form She took in these meditations. Each form that She manifested was self-luminous, radiant in every detail. The clothes She wore, the jewels, necklaces, and bracelets all shone with their own light. In the dark void of meditative awareness, her effulgence was dazzling.

When the first goddess appeared, I was so stunned I didn't know what to do—whether to bow, pray, prostrate, or just tremble in sheer awe. I was simultaneously aware of sitting in the lotus position in meditation next to Baba's chair in the meditation hall in his ashram in New York and being immersed in this meditative vision as it spontaneously unfolded. Suddenly in the vision, an arati tray arrayed with the traditional items—a flame, flowers, rice, turmeric, and gold—appeared in my hands and I knew to do *puja* (ritual of prayer and offering) to Her while She stood inches from me, staring me in the eyes. Oh my God, her eyes . . . if words could only begin to describe their beauty and depth, their love and compassion, their wisdom and joy—and how utterly entrancing they are to gaze into. After a few minutes, I became completely absorbed in Her, dissolving into Her as She embraced me. The drop merged with the ocean. Then the universe disappeared into Her, with all sense of "I" dissolving as well, dissolving into unalloyed ecstasy. After some time, "I" reappeared in the meditation, overwhelmed by love and grace that the union soaked my body and mind with. This sequence repeated itself with each goddess as they appeared in this series of meditative visions.

As I merged with Her in meditation, I felt a total dissolution of the universe; my entire sense of being a person was lost in ecstasy, only reappearing as she gave birth to the universe once again. All through the processes of dissolution and reemergence I could hear her sublime laugh! She totally delighted in creating and dissolving universes within her own being. With generosity so overwhelming as to be literally self-annihilating, she answered my initial prayer to know the highest form of worship of Kundalini. True worship is to merge with the one you worship. Through worship and prayer, Kundalini reveals the mysteries of the universe to the self-disciplined seeker.

The Goddess gave me all the insight and knowledge I needed in order to proceed. If I hoped for Her to reveal more of the divine mystery behind Kundalini awakening and the movement of Shakti up through the chakras, it would be through worshiping Her. I vowed not to do any more work on my dissertation or professional work until I had received some deeper understanding from the Mahadevi (great goddess) Kundalini herself. I stopped all work on my thesis in order to devote my entire attention to the worship of Her. Each morning before meditation, I chanted the Kundalini Stavaha (a beautiful, ancient Sanskrit hymn of praise to Kundalini) and did arati (a traditional Eastern form of worship) to Mahadevi Kundalini. In time She gave me all that I needed, showing me in meditation an allegorical journey symbolic of Kundalini awakening and moving through the subtle body.

JOURNEY BEYOND THE MIND

Through my own experiences and those shared by many people who are deeply engaged in spiritual practices, it is clear that each one of us is on a journey in this life—a journey in which we are propelled toward the further evolution of consciousness, expanding love and compassion, and at a certain stage, Kundalini awakening. In some lives, we might inch forward, and in other lives we might make great leaps. Through the course of my sadhana it became clear to me that as a part of our journey, awakened Kundalini gives us the opportunity to experience all the realms of human existence with extraordinary clarity. We can then recognize their limitations and move on. As Kundalini moves through the chakras, we may be given experiences of them in various bound and constricted states, as well as in purified and expanded states. Kundalini gives each person the experiences they need as they move toward greater and greater freedom. This culminates in the experience of everlasting union with the Infinite and the direct experience of such loving ecstasy that the ego mind is drowned in Love, making it a servant of Love forevermore.

> Though the pages of your life turn
> one day at a time,
> one breath at a time,
> the book of your life is written,
> and it is the book of love.
> Love fills every page,
> every breath.
> All there is
> is Love.
> KALIDAS

Yet if we are blind or unable to read what She has written, then we wander searching for what is already there. By her grace, through awakening, we are able to directly know the eternal truth.

The attainment of the state of union with its boundless love isn't intended to leave one in a disembodied state of transcendence. Instead, this state divinizes our worldly existence. Our Shakti, our power of Consciousness, reemerges from that union transfigured, shining with the Light of Infinite Consciousness, and brings that Light down to earth, down to the realm of the body and mind. As Joseph Campbell makes clear, in all the myths of the hero's journey, the quest isn't complete until the hero returns with the gifts for the rest of humanity. Divine Consciousness "enlightens" the mind and body of saints in this state, the true spiritual heroes who have completed the journey. They glow with this illumination and live only to serve others.

To know and to serve—these are the ultimate purposes of life. Kundalini gives us the gift of knowing who we truly are, of knowing the Divine directly through complete union. Kundalini transforms our instruments of consciousness, the mind and body, so that they may serve through the selfless state of illumination that results from complete transformation.

If you want to progress most rapidly on the journey led by Kundalini, I recommend approaching your sacred Self and its power, Kundalini, with all the reverence and love of which you are capable. And remember that this transformation may take years or even lifetimes. Kundalini remakes and empowers the mind-body instrument to act solely by the promptings of one's divine nature, giving expression to the boundless wisdom, compassion, patience, and love that are your true nature. Kundalini awakening and unfolding allow us to realize the deepest meanings of life and fulfill the greatest purposes of human birth—to know and to serve—regardless of the outer circumstances of our lives.

The great eighteenth-century poet saint of Bengal, Ramprasad Sen wrote:

> Mother of Ultimacy,
> unspeakable and unthinkable,
> who can comprehend your countless revelations?
> Sometimes you remove every veil
>   to be known by enlightened sages

as the formless Mother of the Universe,

the transparent presence who dwells secretly

within every atom, every perception, every event.

Other times you manifest as Mother Kundalini,

the evolutionary potency

coiled at the root of the subtle body.

RAMPRASAD SEN

Whether we call Her Shakti Kundalini, the Great Goddess, Kali, Bhagavati Prajnaparamita, Tara, Holy Mother, or some other name, She bestows the awareness that our body is the body of the universe. Our body is her body. Our awareness encompasses everything from the core of an atom to the grand expanse of the dance of galaxies moving through billions of light-years of space—all of that is within the infinite expanse of Consciousness. That Consciousness is our Being. For this reason, the full realization of Kundalini is beyond the mind; it's beyond anything that the mind can even fantasize. The drop can't contain the ocean; it can't even begin to comprehend the ocean's enormity, though that doesn't stop it from imagining that it does. The mind is of the nature of limited knowing, and so it has to surrender to the fact that direct knowing of that which is unlimited is an experience that lies beyond it. It waits at the gates. It can be informed by it. Our mind can be infused with the boundless love, wisdom, compassion, and awareness that radiates from that direct knowing, which transforms the mind. But that is a precinct of knowing, a domain of knowing, that is beyond the mind. However, it's not beyond knowing, because it's the direct experience of the Infinite that Kundalini bestows. That's why She's known as the power of revelation.

What does She reveal? She reveals the direct experience of who and what we are beyond the mind. She reveals the divine nature of the entire universe and every being within it. Once while I was in meditation, Shakti said, "Look for God, look for your Self, look for the Divine all around you. You already know how to use your eyes for seeing differences, now open your divine sight and see the One appearing as the many." It's the birthright of each and every human being. You are born with the ability; you're born with Kundalini; you just need the right conditions to unfold it. Seek to create the right conditions through prayer, through meditation, through good fellowship, through the company of wise beings, and through a disciplined life.

MEDITATION: KUNDALINI'S EMBRACE:
BECOMING ABSORBED IN THE THROB OF SHAKTI

Meditating on and becoming completely immersed in the maha mantra, the great mantra, Om Namah Shivaya, infuses the meditator with Kundalini's power. Om Namah Shivaya comes through a lineage of masters with fully awakened Kundalini Shakti. It has the power to awaken and carry you forward on the path to radical freedom, to abide in your true nature.

Om Namah Shivaya meditation also clears obstacles from the mind and body, developing greater steadiness. It brings your awareness to the truth of who and what you are, beyond the movements of the mind and body.

Become absorbed in Om Namah Shivaya as you sit now for meditation. Mantra is a vibration of your essential nature. Mantra is unlike any other words or language. It's the full, unimpeded power of consciousness, encoded in sound, in vibration, and in subtler and subtler forms of vibration, until it dissolves into the vibration of light and awareness itself, dissolving the mind and all its thoughts.

Become absorbed in the silent repetition of Om Namah Shivaya, Om Namah Shivaya, allowing the mind to become immersed in that, repeating it over and over within. As the mind becomes more and more absorbed in that inner sound, you may notice that even the subtle, thought-form of the sound of the mantra changes, until there's just a throb or vibration, until there's just a pulse of awareness, of simply being.

You may notice that the mind and thoughts have dissolved; even the thought of mantra has dissolved. You may notice that the mantra has drawn your attention and your awareness to the sacred space of its origin, the source, your own sublime Self, beyond thoughts, beyond words, beyond even the grosser forms of mantra as sound and words.

That bare, spacious awareness, boundless and free, that's the true nature of mantra, that's the true refuge. If the mind arises again with a thought, gently dissolve it once more in Om Namah Shivaya, following it back to that spacious, infinitely free source.

Even after your meditation sitting ends, you can remain in touch with your source by remaining aware of that throb of the mantra, Om Namah Shivaya. The mantra is already vibrating within you. Bringing the mind to the mantra helps to attune the mind to that deeper living presence of wisdom and compassion. The mind can repeat the mantra Om Namah Shivaya at any time and any place throughout the day, to remain collected, to remain free, to delight in the refuge of your own inner Self. In the same way, one can use the mantra Om Kali Ma or the mantras from the Buddhist tradition, Om Mani Padme Hum or Om Tare Tum Soha. These mantras too can serve as a refuge, as a vehicle for drawing the mind back to its source and dissolving the flux of thoughts and feelings, images and memories that occupy the mind. Dissolve them back into that clear spacious awareness.

4

Maps of Kundalini's Domain

The yogic tradition has explored Kundalini's power of Consciousness for literally thousands of years, mapping out the domains She operates within, as well as the structures and dynamics of what is created in the states of consciousness that manifest when Kundalini awakens. Kundalini takes one from a state of being unconscious of and separate from the Divine, as well as separate from the deep meaning and purpose of one's life, through a transformative process that establishes one in a state of intimate knowing of one's unity with the Divine, with everyone, and with the entire world, even while mind and body skillfully function in the everyday world. This ultimate goal of Kundalini unfolding is living *sahaja samadhi,* or living meditation, living in the natural state of being that has transcended and included all the domains of experience. Kundalini transmutes the drives for love, happiness, and freedom by revealing how they are ultimately fulfilled by abiding in one's true nature, embracing and being embraced by the Infinite as one's Self.

The yogic tradition gives us particularly insightful descriptions of how Kundalini's power operates by giving us maps of the spiritual terrain to be crossed on our soul's journey. Maps are representations of actual reality. Just as we now map ocean currents, air currents, even global lines of magnetic power, the ancient sages mapped and passed on to us the structure and dynamics of the subtle body, and they even provide us with a representation of the process by which the Infinite becomes the finite universe. It is these yogic maps that we will explore in this chapter.

THE FIVE POWERS OF THE INFINITE

One of the most beautiful and insightful representations of how the powers of the Divine create our reality comes from the ancient monistic tradition of Kashmir Shaivism. (Remember that even in this sublime tradition, it is the mind, albeit refined and purified, trying to understand and express in words what is completely transcendent. The mind endeavors to make it understandable, both so that it can be informed by that transcendent wisdom arising within, and to try to communicate the experience of merger with the Infinite for the benefit of others.) From the Shaivite perspective God, the Infinite Auspicious One, is said to have five powers, of which everything else in the universe is a manifestation. The power of Shiva (the Auspicious One) is inseparable from its creative power of Consciousness, or Shakti, which holds the five powers: the power to create everything, the power to sustain that creation, the power to destroy everything, the power to conceal anything, and the power to reveal anything, including Her and thus your own Infinite nature. Kashmir Shaivism offers a magnificent map of how we go from being the infinite Shakti/Shiva, boundless in every way imaginable, to being the contracted limited finite form of who we are in this life.

In every moment, these five powers of Shakti/Shiva are manifest, and we can see them at play in our own mind. Our mind reflects the operation of these five powers within the contracted domain of our little universe of personal experience. We have all the powers of the Infinite, only in diminished forms. We create something in our mind, and then we hold it there and sustain it for as long as we want. We then dissolve that form and get rid of it, or we might conceal it and tuck it away in our memory, revealing it again by bringing it back to conscious awareness. In this way, the ordinary mind is constantly reflecting these five infinite powers of our divine nature, but in a limited form.

FIVE POWERS EXERCISE

Knowing yourself as Shakti/Shiva playing with your five magnificent powers is as easy as taking a moment now to watch the play of your powers unfolding in the spacious awareness of your mind.

You have the power to create, sustain, dissolve, conceal, and reveal right now, right here. Take a moment to watch your mind and label each of these powers in action.

You might close your eyes for a few moments or gaze off into space as you turn your attention to the inner space, the inner sky of awareness, and watch what you create. Thoughts and images, memories and sensations, arise, are sustained, dissolve, are concealed in your memory, or are revealed by bringing them back to awareness.

Keep watching with detached wonder at the play of your own powers. You are also creating the experience of being a limited form of Shakti/Shiva, playing in the sandbox of your mind, while your fully expanded Shakti/Shiva nature watches with pure joy, unbounded ecstasy!

Delight in this as long as you like. You can come back to this awareness at any time in any place, even as the mind engages in what it needs to do in the moment.

What's very interesting and insightful for understanding Kundalini is that the power of revelation is innate, and the process of Kundalini awakening unfolds this innate capacity. Kundalini reveals what the power of concealment has hidden—our unity with the Divine. This power is also known as *Maya Shakti,* the power to create limitation. The Infinite is boundless; that's what it means to be infinite. *Maya* means "measurable" so it's by the use of the Infinite's own power, Maya Shakti, that it takes on the limitations inherent to all forms—the immeasurable becomes measurable, the Infinite becomes finite, the One becomes many by its own choice. You've chosen to take on the limitations of mind and body. Just as it takes the use of the Auspicious One's power to create the illusion of separation and limitation, it takes the use of the Auspicious One's power of revelation to dispel that illusion. The mind alone will never accomplish this.

This map is another extraordinary illumination of how the unimpeded power of the Infinite takes on innumerable finite forms, which it then comes to know by inhabiting them, entering into them with consciousness. First Shakti has to conceal its own infinitude from itself. The Infinite won't fit in the finite unless it willingly takes on that limitation. This isn't true of just heralded manifestations of the Divine—such as Jesus, Buddha, or Krishna. This taking on of limitation is true of every form—from the electrons in the atoms making up this word to the entire cosmos. On an individual level the power of concealment allows one to have the conscious experience of limitations and separation, the boundaries of "I am a man" or "I am a woman" or "I am a child" or whatever limited container "I" consciousness enters through identification. Unlimited "I-Consciousness" is our Infinite nature. The power of concealment allows it to know the limitations of the finite universe it creates. Your ordinary finite self, who you've always thought yourself to be, is the Divine knowing what it is to be you, choosing to be you as you.

Kundalini as the power of grace, the power of revelation, reverses the power of concealment. The goal of Kundalini awakening is the full and complete experience of our self and the entire world at one with the Divine. Full and complete Kundalini awakening is the Divine choosing to know Itself simultaneously as finite and Infinite.

THE THREE MALAS COVERING OUR INFINITE NATURE

When the Infinite, which has become a limited being, wants to know itself as the Godhead, as Shakti/Shiva once again, it exercises its power of revelation. Kundalini, as I've mentioned, is that power. It brings us back to the infinite expanse and play of our powers of consciousness. It enables us to see our powers of consciousness operating moment by moment and know we are creating the reality we experience. Shaktipat, the descent of grace that awakens Kundalini, is what cuts through the root cause of why consciousness has become bound. In Kashmir Shaivism, the root cause of this bondage is called *anava mala*. A *mala* is a covering or cloak that hides our true nature. Anava mala is the putting on of the cloak of ignorance, or *avidya,* the primal ignorance of not knowing our Self, of not knowing that we are the Infinite, and of not knowing our Buddha-mind or Christ-consciousness. The power of concealment hides the very truth of our boundless nature. In order to create the universe of limited forms, the Infinite has to be able to say in a sense, "I am not the Infinite," "I am not Buddha," which sets the stage for limited individual consciousness to emerge: "I am a suffering being caught in endless cycles of birth and death." It's taking on that limitation, anava mala, which gives us the experience of the limited being we've become.

Consciousness has to leave the reality of radically free Infinite Being to enter the theater of limited individuality. That's where the drama of life unfolds with all its transient pleasures and suffering. Kashmir Shaivism describes two additional malas that further obscure our original nature. *Mayiya mala* creates the subtle and physical bodies, limiting consciousness to them. *Karma mala* binds consciousness to the impressions left by actions and desires arising in the subtle and physical bodies. Covered by the malas, we're bound within the fleeting nature of time as we briefly flash into and out of existence, clinging to all we cherish, creating life after life driven by lacking this and wanting that. The malas are a representation or map of how the illusion of separate existence comes into reality.

CONTEMPLATION

To get a better understanding of this process, imagine a vast deep ocean, calm and still, as the Infinite Consciousness of the Divine. God begins to create and a wave forms on the ocean, a form that seems to have its individual existence, yet is still one with the ocean. Now imagine that the wave's oneness with the ocean is concealed from it, and the wave is given permission to play at taking on all different kinds of forms. The wave as a wave of Consciousness is conscious itself in a limited way and experiences itself as a huge wave, then a small wave, a ripple, a tall wave, a fat wave, and on and on. Shedding one form and taking on another. But, as with all activities, this gets boring after a while. The wave has learned all it could from taking on different shapes, and now it's no longer creative or meaningful to continue doing it. The wave has a vague memory of having been a part of something greater and begins to long for something greater. It wants to reunite with the ocean, with God. This is where the fifth power of God comes in, the power of grace, the power of revelation. By an act of grace, God undoes the work of its own power of concealment and reveals the truth of the unbroken unity with God. The wave delights in being a projection of the ocean. The illusion of separation is dissolved and once again it knows the ecstasy of oneness with our Creator.

The fifteenth-century poet Saint Kabir, reflecting on this illusion, wrote:

> Rising, water's still water,
> falling back, it is water,
> will you give me a hint
> how to tell them apart?[1]

The descriptions of the five-fold power of Shakti Kundalini and the way the malas conceal our true infinite nature empower us with the insight needed to see through the blinding details of all the forms arising in the mind and the world. Regaining the perspective of our Self, of Shakti Kundalini, we can see the magnificent dynamics of creation unfolding, manifesting all these forms out of the one essence, Shakti. It's like walking through a huge jewelry store and seeing all the gold necklaces, gold bracelets, rings, charms, earrings, and on and on. Then stepping back and seeing all the gold, in all the display cases, sparkling in different shapes and forms and uses, while remaining, simply, gold. There is nothing that is not Shakti Kundalini!

THE COILED SERPENT: SYMBOL OF THE DIVINE WITHIN

As I've mentioned, the power of Kundalini is fully present in everyone, but in most people it lies inactive, dormant, until the great awakening that marks the most sacred event in the soul's journey back to its source. Kundalini is often symbolically depicted in yogic texts as a coiled serpent lying asleep within us, a serpent whose mighty powers become manifest as it awakens and uncoils. In meditation, one might even see the archetypal form of a coiled snake that gives Kundalini its name. The ancient symbol of the snake, a symbol of the Divine Feminine, and the lingam, a symbol of the Divine Masculine, around which the snake is wrapped, are visual forms that the Infinite as Shakti/Shiva takes on in the base chakra, the muladhara. The snake and the lingam depict the divine union of feminine and masculine, Holy Mother and Holy Father, as fully present throughout creation—from the infinitely expanded formless, transcendent realm of the sahasrara (crown chakra) to the earth realm of bound forms in the muladhara. All of this lies within you right now.

This may sound unbelievable, or just too fantastic! But what if I were to tell you it's a well-researched fact that within each person there is a spiral form of bound energy that holds more knowledge than the world's best scientists can comprehend.

This spiral form of bound energy awakens and begins to unfold its unfathomable intelligence when the two halves of the spiral are joined to form a whole.

You can't see this coiled form of bound energy inside you. It's microscopic in size, and yet it knows how to grow an entire human being from a single cell. It guided the development of one infinitesimally small bit of protoplasm into all the trillions of different cells that make up your body. This spiral form of bound energy knew how to transform that one microscopic speck of living substance into your heart, lungs, nerves, brain, eyes, ears, nose, skin, teeth, bones, and muscles. It knew how to create all the different cells—white blood cells, red blood cells, nerve and muscle cells, bone and cartilage cells. It knew where to grow them and when to stop growing them. It lets your fingernails grow but not your fingers; it lets your hair grow but not your ears; it grew your heart in the right place and connected it to your head. It knew where to grow each artery and vein in your entire circulatory system. It knew just the right place to grow the nerve cells that run all the way from your big toe up to your brain and back again.

Does this sound too incredible? Do I really expect you to believe that a microscopic, spiral form of bound energy knows how to do all that? Yes! We don't know how, but we do know that DNA, the spiral form of bound energy that makes up your genes, guides the truly miraculous development of a single cell into the unimaginably complex organization of trillions of cells, which we call the human body. If the energy of the universe can be bound in the molecules forming DNA, subtly encoding in it all the information necessary to create from itself the many diverse organs, tissues, and cells of the body and have them successfully operate together, what makes you think a little Consciousness couldn't be lying dormant within you, symbolized as a coiled serpent, waiting to propel your awareness back to union with the Creator? DNA isn't Kundalini, but it serves to demonstrate how a vast amount of information—the organization and functioning of every cell and even the biochemistry within trillions of cells—can be packed into something so tiny it is seemingly imperceptible, invisible to the naked eye. Kundalini is there within you even if you don't yet perceive that power. Perhaps She has already begun to stir from her slumber!

THE SOUL'S EVOLUTION ACROSS LIFETIMES

What is that process of consciousness evolving, and what is the soul learning across countless lifetimes through many life-forms? In the yogic tradition the evolution of consciousness occurs over countless lifetimes and encompasses incarnations in many different life-forms. The yogic tradition also provides a map or representation of how that process of evolution unfolds. One way of understanding this is to look at a circle and imagine the circular pattern as the soul's process of learning across numerous lifetimes. The following diagram depicts this.

You can see that the right half of the circle proceeds through the process of involution. This "outgoing phase" is called *savritti* (from twelve o'clock to six

FIGURE 1 EVOLUTION OF CONSCIOUSNESS ACROSS LIFETIMES

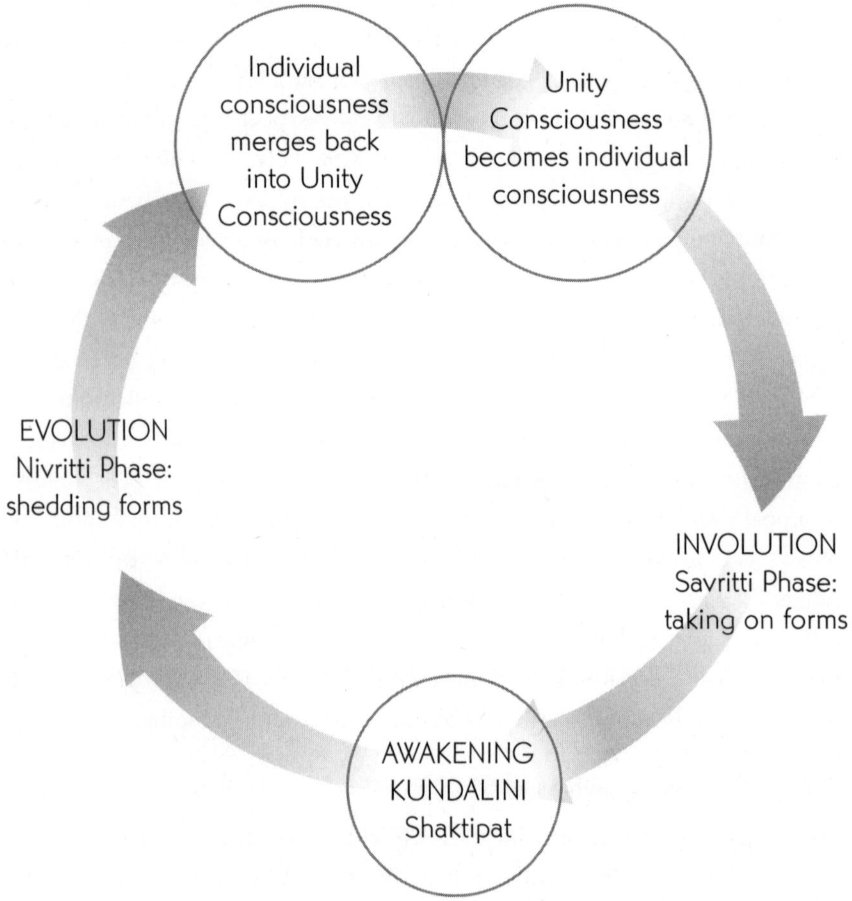

o'clock), and the "return phase" (from six back to twelve) is *nivritti*. The savritti part of the cycle is where the soul or consciousness is developing through involution, taking on forms. It is exploring what it is to be an individualized consciousness, going through all the many countless incarnations, learning from each one of them about the consequences of its own actions, the causes of suffering, the power of love, the dynamics of creation, and on and on. It is experiencing all the different things that we can encounter in life after life after life. The second half of the journey, nivritti, symbolizes the development that occurs through shedding forms. This is the release, the letting go of identification with bound structures, the clearing out of karmas while endeavoring to create as little new karma as possible and only positive karma at that. The nivritti phase begins with the first stirrings of Kundalini and continues until consciousness regains the fullness of its true boundless nature in a living state of radical freedom, living samadhi. The savritti-nivritti cycle maps out the evolution of the soul across countless lives.

There comes a point near the end of the savritti phase where the soul says to itself, "I've learned enough; I've been through the countless cycles of birth and death; I've learned so many things through that, but the suffering is wearisome. The lack of true freedom is too confining. The lasting fullness, unbreakable joy, the boundless love I seek will never be gained in this manner." At this point the soul is intuiting that there's much more to life. There's much more to who and what we are than living within the confines of a mind and a body, the confines of identification with being a man or a woman, young or old, all those different aspects that we take for granted as defining who we are. We begin to recognize that no matter how much we own and consume, joy is fleeting, power is temporary, and old age, decline, and death are inevitable. We begin to intuit that there was an original experience of being connected with something deeper, eternal, ecstatic, and serene. How can we regain that?

That time of awakening is the point in the soul's evolutionary cycle between going out to explore all that occurs with contracting and taking on forms and the return part of the cycle where the soul goes through the process of expansion and shedding forms. It is at this time in the cycle that we summon our innate power to know the Self to arise again. It's the time for the descent of grace, for Holy Spirit to baptize the soul anew, for bodhicitta to ascend and outshine the conditioned mind; it is time for the most auspicious event—shaktipat.

Shaktipat is often symbolized as a lightning bolt, and just as lightning only strikes the ground when there is a charge built up in the earth below as well as in the sky above, in the ground of our soul we build the charge of seeking to be free of the endless death and rebirth cycles that go with the savritti phase.

That entire cycle of taking on forms and then relinquishing them isn't just the cycle that plays out across countless lifetimes; it's also a cycle that occurs within each life. Look at what happens from the time we're born until we mature and go through old age and death: notice the vast amount of growth and change, expansion and contraction, that occurs as we're trying on different identities—first as an infant, then as a child, then an adolescent, then as a student, as an employee, in relationships. Within each life we might explore what it is to be a husband, a wife, or a partner, a father or a mother. We explore what happens to our consciousness as it fills the container of identity associated with those different roles. As we mature with those roles and identities, there inevitably comes the time later in life when we start to step back from them. Some fall away with age. For example, we have to stop being an adolescent and become an adult, or we graduate from school, get fired, get divorced, or have an accident or disease that robs us of functioning. We're left with no choice but to let go of some identities, until finally at death, we shed even the body. That same kind of process, that same arc of development that involves taking on forms of our own creation and dissolving them, goes across each lifetime that we experience.

The same kind of cycle repeats itself every day. You wake up in the morning and literally start to take on roles. You might begin your day by thinking, "What do I have to do today?" and you put on the role of your work. Maybe it's a day off, "Oh, what am I going to do with my children, or with my spouse, or by myself?" We put on a different role for each relationship, a different identity, or a different facet of our identity. We might even put on the clothes that go with that role identity. If we're going to work, we might have the uniform that goes with work, whether it's a suit and tie or a different kind of uniform associated with that role. As we put it on, we assume that role and our consciousness enters it and we have the experience of entering into that role. "I am _____" is the thought-form that goes with this process of identification, the process of consciousness pouring itself into the containers: I am a professional, I am unemployed, I am a mother, I am a man, I am a woman, and on and on. We go through the whole day in this manner, and then there comes a time later in the day when it's time to start shedding those roles, shedding those identities. Maybe we do it on the way home, maybe we do it when we walk to our bedroom and take off the uniform that we had on during the day and put on something that's light and comfortable.

When the day finally comes to an end, we put on the clothes for sleep, another symbolic change in uniforms. And we have to literally shed and drop all those roles and identities in order to be able to shift from that ordinary waking state into the sleep state. In fact, if we're not able to shed all of our daily roles, it may prevent us from being able to fall asleep. We may be stressed, we may be agitated, or we might be excited. We might have to do something to let go of the day and all we took on, to shift states and go into deep sleep. In the dire circumstance where we can't let go, where the conditioned mind is so identified and clinging to the things of the day, where the brain won't disengage, we may even resort to medications to wipe away the waking state mind and clear all the enervation that comes from identifying with this or that role. What we're seeking is freedom from the confines and stresses of the forms we've taken on all day, like the savritti phase of involution coming to completion and the nivritti phase of letting go, leading us to greater peace and contentment. However, with ordinary sleep the expanded consciousness of awakened Kundalini isn't present, the relief is fleeting, and the next morning we continue on the treadmill, chasing effervescent joys and dreams, taking on limited identities to engage in their pursuit. Kundalini awakening leads to the state of radical freedom that already lies waiting for you, just beyond deep sleep and the dreamlike existence of the ordinary mind.

AWAKENING

The analogy of waking from sleep is a good way to understand the process of what happens when Kundalini becomes active. Imagine you are sound asleep; the alarm goes off or the dog jumps on the bed and suddenly you've gone from one reality—the reality of a deep sleep or a dream—to the waking state reality of lying in your bed. You discover that you've woken up to what was already fully present, the world around you, but now you're awake and aware and experiencing it directly. One moment you can be in a dream reality and the next moment awaken to the everyday reality of your waking world, which was already fully present but you were unconscious of it during your deep sleep or dreams. Kundalini awakening empowers us to directly know the presence that already is here—the Divine, the Infinite presence that already fully exists. It's not suddenly created; we're simply and profoundly waking up to it, to our unbroken union with God. Though awakening is a metaphor, it is useful because it provides a representation, a map, of the process of going from the limited state of unconsciousness or dreams to a state of consciousness in which we recognize what was already fully present.

Directly knowing our intimate connection with every human being, our intimate connection with nature, and our sense of unity with All are some ways that the experience of awakening may reveal itself. For some people, awakening happens walking in the woods and suddenly feeling a profound connectedness to every living presence there, trees, shrubs, birds, bugs, or even the rocks. For another person, this sense of connection might occur when they were in the middle of Grand Central Station; suddenly the quality of sound, the vitality of people, and everything around them is part of their awakened experience of being at one with the flow of all of that life, all of that hustle and bustle, all of the universes that each and every person represents—their suffering, their pains, their longings, their happiness, and their intimate connection with all that.

By entering into meditative states, we get to merge with that Source consciously, freeing ourselves from the ordinary ego mind. The innate power that allows us to do that is Kundalini Shakti, the power of Consciousness that can transform and inform the entirety of our waking state life and our dream worlds as well. Then we are empowered to wake up to our true Self, our true nature, and go through our day-to-day activities from an entirely different level of consciousness, with the ego mind informed by the fullness of our Infinite nature, imbued with boundless patience, wisdom, love, and compassion for all.

The ordinary ego mind has to be closed to the Infinitude in order to function in waking state reality. That's its job. If someone doesn't recognize boundaries and limitations in their everyday functioning, then they will be diagnosed with a mental illness. A healthy ego mind isn't the problem; it's the conditioned, habitual identification with just the ego mind that separates us experientially from the boundlessness of our original Being and drives the ego mind to act in ignorance of the sublime nature of the world, others, and ourselves—all united in Being. The uninformed ego mind goes from one state of lack and want to momentary satisfactions and then onto the next state of lack and want. Only by coming to rest in the infinite fullness of your true nature can you abide in peace, contentment, and ecstasy. Only then are you radically free, fully awake, a Buddha, a Knower, a tathagata, one who has gone beyond.

Kundalini creates the vehicles of mind and body and inhabits them for countless cycles of birth and death, exploring all that can be known through them of the joys and pains of everyday life. Kundalini also creates the path to regaining the Unity Consciousness that puts out the fires of suffering and craving, extinguishing them in an ocean of love and ecstasy. Then the mind and body are moved by wisdom and true knowledge instead of ignorance and endless cravings. The same vehicles of the mind/subtle body and the physical body can serve either ignorance and cravings or wisdom and love. Kundalini empowers you to choose wisely.

KUNDALINI: SOURCE OF THE CAUSAL, SUBTLE, AND PHYSICAL BODIES

The yogic tradition maps many details of how the Infinite becomes the finite physical world of forms, such as the human body itself. As discussed earlier, it begins with the negation of Unity Consciousness, the negation of infinite power and eternal existence through the five powers and the imposition of the three malas, or coverings. This initial negation of infinitude creates the bound space and time within which creation proceeds. That bound space and time where our Infinitude has been negated, but the multiplicity of finite forms has yet to arise, is called the *causal body.* Aptly named due to it causing all that follows: the creation of countless forms and the desires, the motive force behind creation, of seeking what was lost. The causal body is experienced in deep sleep as the continuous awareness of nothingness. The light of the Infinite has been negated and no forms have yet evolved. The black void of deep sleep reflects this state of no-thingness, no forms have emerged for the mind to perceive. The subtle seed of limited I-awareness is present, but insufficient consciousness is there to perceive it. All the ordinary mind knows of the causal state of deep sleep is that there is a thread of the sense of self that continues through the unconsciousness of that state. When by Kundalini's grace one visits this state in meditation, it will become clearer.

Out of the causal body arises the subtle body, which I mentioned earlier and is created by Shakti Kundalini to serve as a vehicle for experiencing limitations, desires, actions, and all the lessons that consciousness will evolve through over the course of innumerable lifetimes. Dream sleep is the state in which the ordinary mind most fully experiences the subtle body. In meditation, Kundalini can illumine the subtle body more fully than the ordinary mind can with its limited light of consciousness. The subtle body creates the physical body. Each of the physical senses as well as the physical organs has its origin in a principle constituent of the subtle body.

Within the subtle body along the sushumna nadi are the chakras, or the operating centers of consciousness. The chakras are situated along the sushumna nadi at intersections of lesser nadis, similar to the nerve centers along the spinal cord.

Chakra is a Sanskrit word that means "circle" or "wheel;" it's the root of the English words *circus* and *circle*. The chakras may appear to the inner eye during meditation as wheels of energy or light, and they are also described as lotus flowers with various numbers of petals. The energy channels intersecting at a chakra form what appear to be the petals of a flower. The highest center, technically not a chakra though it is commonly referred to as one, is the thousand-petaled lotus of the sahasrara. Because the energy in the subtle body is conscious energy, these energy centers are actually operating centers of consciousness. The descent of Consciousness from the sahasrara, the transcendent domain of pure Consciousness above the sushumna nadi to the energy center at the base, called the *muladhara,* the earth realm, marks the process of consciousness going from the highest transcendent Unity Consciousness to the limitations of embodied consciousness that you and I normally experience as we live out our existence in the world.

The muladhara chakra represents the element of earth and is the final destination of Divine Consciousness, Kundalini Shakti, through the process of descent and manifestation of the world. It is within this chakra that Kundalini lies dormant after creating the world and embodied existence. It is here that She awaits the Great Awakening that will reverse this process, removing the limitations consciousness has taken on and allowing us to once again be aware of our transcendent, unbounded, divine nature, as the wave merges back into the sea.

The process of involution is that of consciousness descending from the formless transcendent Godhead, condensing to the earthly realm of human existence. Evolution reverses this, with consciousness ascending back up through the chakras, becoming ever freer of limitations, restrictions, and the illusion of being bound and separate from its source—God/Goddess.

In descending order the seven major chakras are: the sahasrara at the crown of the head, the ajna chakra between the eyes, the vishuddha chakra in the throat, the anahata chakra near the heart, the manipura chakra at about the level of the solar plexus, the svadhishthana chakra at the root of the sexual organs, and the muladhara chakra at the base of the pelvis. The involution of consciousness from the transcendent realm of the sahasrara on down to the muladhara is in part symbolized in the progressive order of the elements that each chakra represents. Involution is a process of consciousness coalescing, becoming grosser, denser, and more limited.

Just below the sahasrara is the ajna chakra, the "third eye," between and above our physical eyes, and this is the realm of pure individualized mind. Consciousness at this level has lost its formless, all-encompassing universality but hasn't yet coalesced into the physical realm. Here consciousness may be experienced simply as a limited sense of "I-ness" that doesn't yet have all the qualities we normally experience as ourselves, like our gender, body shape, and role.

The subsequent five chakras represent the manifestation of the five elements comprising the physical realm, along with increasingly contracted states of consciousness, emotional patterns, and more. These subtle body centers contain the subtle elements that create the entire human body. They aren't the physical elements themselves, but the subtle energy principle underlying the physical reality of these elements: space, air, fire, water, earth. The subtle body is entirely comprised of subtle energies—there are no gross physical components to it, nothing measurable by physical instruments, which frustrate scientific efforts to research the subtle body. Only correlates of its activity reflected in changes of the physical body can be measured. However, yogis, researchers of the inner worlds, refined their consciousness through meditation and the grace of Kundalini Shakti. They were and are able to directly perceive and map the subtle body. You have the same innate capability, though exploring the subtle body is not necessary and may even be a distraction from reaching the goal of Kundalini unfolding.

In descending order, there is a progression from the subtlest to the grossest of the elements. Just looking at the elements, the next chakra, the vishuddha, at the level of the throat, represents the element of ether or space, the subtlest of the physical elements. After this we descend to the anahata chakra, the heart chakra and the element of air, as consciousness becomes a bit denser and grosser than it was at the level symbolized by space. Next is the manipura chakra with the element of fire. Fire is still subtle, but it has more definition and is grosser than air. The svadhishthana chakra, which represents the element water, comes next. Water is denser and more substantial than fire but not as gross and dense as earth, the last element, which is associated with the muladhara chakra at the base of the sushumna nadi. At this level we've come to the densest, grossest, most limited and bound form of consciousness, the earthly physical realm.

FIGURE 2 THE PRINCIPLE CHAKRAS OF THE SUBTLE BODY

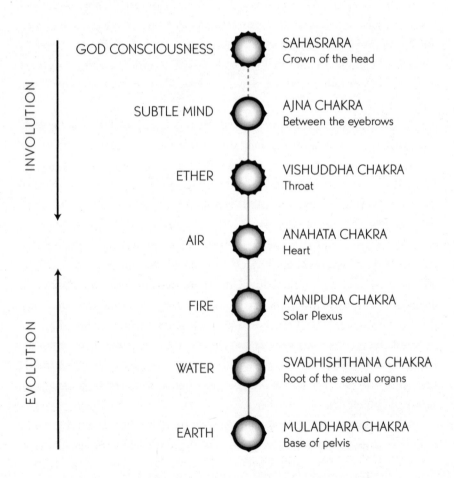

Thus everything from the most subtle sense of Infinite I-awareness to the physical domain of earthly matter is made of consciousness in varying levels of contraction. Even within the most bound forms of the physical realm, the full power and presence of God, of Divine Consciousness, are present. The release of that bound energy is like the release of the potential energy bound in matter that suddenly results in the extraordinary power and light of nuclear reactions. The awakening of Kundalini is the release of the bound power and light of the Divine present within the human form.

When Kundalini awakens—in other words, when our ability to move our awareness beyond the limitations of body and mind comes to life—the energy of Consciousness, also called Shakti, moves up the sushumna nadi and pierces the chakras in ascending order, though it can reverse order and revisit chakras repeatedly, in any order, during the process of clearing out bound patterns of energy and consciousness. Overall, Consciousness as Kundalini Shakti moves from the solid confines of the earth realm, ever expanding, shedding limitations along the way until it finally reaches the unbounded realm of the sahasrara once again. The finite once again knows its union with the Infinite, and we experience reunion with the Divine, the Self of All. The final stages happen beyond the mind, beyond words, beyond the ability of mind and words to encode that experience and speak of it. The fullness of Being is known in silence.

If you were going to navigate your way across the Pacific Ocean, you would want maps that show ocean depths and where mountains rise from the sea floor to form islands. You would need to know where the dangerous reefs are that hide below the waves, threatening your safe voyage. You would want maps of sea currents and prevailing winds, and of course, you would want someone who has been across and back to help you navigate. The maps that sages and yogis brought back from crossing the ocean of samsara, of delusion and ignorance, to help others to cross safely are what we have in the depictions of the five powers, the malas, and the bodies—causal, subtle, and gross—representing the condensing and contracting of the Infinite One to form the manifold finite forms of the gross body. Awakened Kundalini empowers us to see that fully, to delight in all of it as our own Self and regain the direct experience of our ever-present, never broken, all-encompassing wholeness. Maps such as the ones of the chakras, nadis, and the subtle body help to guide us on the journey to fully expanded consciousness.

DECODING THE SYMBOLS IN KUNDALINI'S MAPS

There's much more to the chakras and what they symbolize than the brief description I offer in this book. Each is a level of consciousness, and the yogic sages have explored and given detailed accounts of each of them. Each chakra has associated with it certain powers and characteristic feelings that affect how we create our individual reality—our relationships, our worldview, our sense of self, and our ways of interacting with the world—when we are acting predominantly from the level of that chakra. The petals of each chakra vibrate with a specific letter of the Sanskrit alphabet, and if you add up all the petals from the muladhara to the ajna chakra you get the fifty letters of the alphabet. There's a bija mantra, a seed mantra or syllable, that goes with each chakra, and on and on, layer after layer of details and symbols, all mapping out how the power of Consciousness, Kundalini, creates the microcosm of your limited mind-body self. If you read Sir John Woodroffe's book *Serpent Power,* which includes translations of the yogic texts dealing with all the chakras and Kundalini, you'll be awed by the rich symbolism and the extraordinary map of Consciousness they provide.

It is imperative to remember that even the best of maps isn't the terrain itself. This is even more evident with symbolic maps. The subtle body map is a highly symbolic map of consciousness depicting the chakras as centers of consciousness, root energies of elements and organs of the physical body, and the like in mandala form. It's important to understand the symbolic nature of these depictions, especially because now what's being written about Kundalini, chakras, nadis, and so forth, whether in books or on websites, makes this all look very concrete, as if you could just visualize these descriptions and you've got it. Why would yogis do intense sadhana practices for lifetimes to be able to experience these things if direct knowledge could be had so easily?

Chakras may be depicted in very concrete forms as a lotus of so many petals, but the actual chakras are not concrete physical expressions of the power of Consciousness, Kundalini Shakti. Chakras are a rich mix of consciousness, symbols, and subtle energies outside of the physical realm. Nothing about a chakra is concrete. It's very important to understand the difference between concrete forms and symbols.

Symbols point beyond themselves and have been used for thousands of years in myths, religions, shamanic traditions, and other esoteric traditions like the Masons and Kabbalistic teachings to transmit teachings, power, and energy and to protect teachings and practices from the uninitiated. A symbol may be used to point to a state of consciousness, a teaching, process, or even a passageway that can't be exactly expressed in words. This can be something as simple as a black dot—a point that's called the *bindu* that is often at the center of a *yantra* (a complex visual symbol used for entering certain meditations). That bindu is a symbol of the portal through which consciousness has to go in order to move beyond even the symbolic realm into the infinite expanse that goes beyond words, the mind, and what even a symbol can point to. But if we mistake a symbol for a sign, for example thinking, "There's a six-pointed star, that's Jewish," then it's just a sign, and one loses the meaning of the downward pointing triangle as symbolic of the Divine Feminine and the upward pointing triangle as symbolic of the Divine Masculine with the combination symbolizing the Divine union present throughout creation (a symbol of that union which you'll find in yantras and in chakras). It is not just a sign of the Jewish tradition. It has deep symbolic meaning within the Jewish tradition and beyond it.

When we encounter all these extraordinary symbols and the symbolic maps of consciousness as we explore the depths of Kundalini, it is important that we remember these are highly symbolic representations of Consciousness taking on form. In the Zen tradition, they very simply say, "Don't confuse the finger for the moon." The finger points at the moon, but it's not the moon. Teachings, concepts, and symbols all may point to the full light of Consciousness, but they aren't it. A symbol points to something beyond itself; it's not that thing. Simply grasping the teaching, the concept, the symbol, doesn't give one the moon.

It's that form of symbolic thinking that is also important for understanding these maps. Sages and seers express things symbolically because it is also a way of protecting those teachings. The symbolically encoded teachings are referred to as *self-protecting* because the power and truth of the teachings are embedded in symbols that an uninitiated person can't grasp. All their concrete thinking about it, regardless of how many years or lifetimes they pursue it, will never unfold the power that the symbol is pointing to. It's part of why it has always been important that one study with someone who truly knows the teachings, truly experiences them, and can pass on all that lies beyond the symbol, beyond what one might find in a book or scripture, or find on the Internet. For this reason many traditions have formalized the practice of passing on the power necessary to truly receive the teachings. In Tibetan Buddhism, empowerments are given ritually and symbolically before the teachings, precisely because without the empowerment, the teachings won't be fully understood and won't have full potency.

Typically, our ordinary mind approaches things with the hubris of the ego. The ego is just going to go after what it wants no matter what. It doesn't even consider an approach of humility and reverence, an approach of devotion. But the best way to receive the great gifts that Kundalini has to bestow is to approach Her with reverence and humbly receive *all* her gifts—whatever they may be. It takes trust and faith. That lesson is often one that the ego mind has a hard time with regardless of whether it is approaching Kundalini for the first time or has already been on Kundalini's path for years. If you want to draw close to someone, love is the way. Approach the Divine within you with love, cherish her gifts with love, merge in Her through love.

5

The Ego and the Self

The ego mind is identified with and attached to being in charge of its domain, especially its inner world. This isn't true for just control freaks! We have led our entire lives with a sense of our "me," our sense of "I-ness." We aim to stay in control or to gain control. The ego mind is the individualized experience of dominator mode consciousness. We wake up in the morning saying, "Oh, I want to do this today. I want to do that. I'd like to accomplish this. I have to deal with that." It's all, "I, I, I, me, me, me, mine, mine, mine, what am I after, what do I want, what will I get out of this." This is what the ego mind does all the time. The ego mind structure evolved for predication and control to serve our survival and procreation instincts. It is very skilled at this. That's good. The yogic and meditative traditions assume a healthy functioning ego as a baseline for engaging in sadhana, though that's not always the case. It takes a dedicated ego and a surrendered ego to get up early in the morning and do all of one's practices before entering the day and fulfilling all one's responsibilities to one's family, work, and community, while remaining mindful of one's practices, contemplations, and practice of selflessness throughout every moment of the day, and finally ending the day with additional practices. The path includes everything in our lives and the ego mind has its rightful place in sadhana.

Often what's most challenging for people when they begin to have experiences of Kundalini processes is that the ego mind struggles with the shift from believing it is in charge of one's life to suddenly confronting the fact that there is this innate other power taking charge. Sometimes people don't know it is the power of their own Divine Self, and even if they do, the ego mind has to work to develop deeper and deeper levels of understanding and surrender, as well as strength, in order to receive all that is being offered by Kundalini. If the ego mind becomes overwhelmed and loses its ability to function, it can require professional mental health care to re-stabilize it. We don't yet have a Kundalini retreat setting to help people through such challenging periods of Kundalini activity. There really aren't any "centers" that offer the mentoring and courses on Kundalini's sublime yoga that will help to ease people through this extraordinary process.

With the shift in consciousness from ego dominance to emerging Universal Consciousness, we evolve entirely different ways of relating to our self, others, and the world. That's a huge set of changes for the ego mind. It can take years and years for the ego mind to integrate experiences and be fully transformed by them. This is simply part of the transformation process of Kundalini awakening one to her reality, her world, the world of your Self. In time, the ego mind becomes the servant of the Self, of the Divine within, instead of a pseudo-master who really is the servant of instincts, family, or cultural expectations and habits of the conditioned, deluded mind. Until we are free from the mind's deluded state, we will continue to experience endless rounds of birth, suffering, and death.

Kundalini, the power of the infinite that literally creates the universe, including the mind, the ego, the body, and everything else, invites us to know our Self as the Creator. She invites us to know our Self as creation, to know our Self as every creature, and to know our Self as the very process of creation. We encompass them all. The creature of the ego, the creature of our own life, the embodied one going through whatever we are going through, is but one tiny aspect of our total Consciousness. The ego mind isn't separate from Kundalini anymore than your hand is separate from your body. There's often a longing in us to know something greater than our self, to go beyond what the ordinary mind is seeking. That may be an initial stirring of Kundalini in the form of the longing to return, to wake up, to go beyond the wearisome contracted states of mind-body awareness.

We frequently have to remember that Kundalini is an innate power. The ego mind often relates to it as something foreign, something different, even something alien—but it is more you, in fact, than your ego mind. Kundalini with its boundless Consciousness is more truly who you are than anything you think yourself to be. Coming to know that is the grace of Kundalini. Kundalini is stirring as you begin to awaken to the facts that you have a mind, but you're not your mind; that you have thoughts, but you are not your thoughts; that you have feelings, but you're not your feelings; that you have a body, but you're not your body. The relationships that you're in, the things that you've done, don't define or bind the real you. The Infinite Consciousness that becomes all those things and that is truly who you are is your true nature, and knowing this is the gift of Kundalini. By knowing the truth of your Divine nature, you are empowered to go back into all the roles that you play, the relationships that you're in, the things that you do in your everyday life—but now you're informed by this magnificent Consciousness of the truth of who and what you are, as well as the truth of the Divine nature of each and every person you look at. Seeing the beauty, the divinity, the sublime nature of every person, everything that you encounter, is the gift of grace, the awakening of this power of Consciousness that is you.

VARIETIES OF KUNDALINI AWAKENING

Just as the Divine has two aspects, the transcendent and the imminent, Kundalini does as well. One aspect is already fully awake and functioning—that's the imminent aspect that created the body and keeps it going; every beat of your heart, every inhalation and exhalation is happening by the power of Kundalini to sustain the physical body. It is this aspect of Kundalini that is the mind. Every thought is a form of that energy, of Shakti, of Kundalini, that takes the form of a feeling, a thought, a sensation, a memory, a dream. All of those are forms of Kundalini purposely created by binding the power of Consciousness into those forms. But typically the imminent aspect of Kundalini that is sustaining the body, the functioning of the mind and everyday life, is not what is referred to as Kundalini. It's the dormant transcendent aspect, the power of Infinite Consciousness, the illuminating and transforming power of Shakti, that's referred to by the term Kundalini. It's the awakening of that power that initiates the transformative processes of Kundalini unfolding.

As mentioned earlier, Kundalini awakening can happen in a number of ways. Shaktipat literally means "descent of grace, descent of power" and refers to an influx of conscious power, Shakti, that leads to the enlivening, the awakening of Kundalini out of its dormant state into an active state. And that awakening, that descent of grace, has been recognized in many different traditions—in the Christian tradition it's often symbolized by a dove, and the dove is a symbol of the Holy Spirit descending on someone or as part of being baptized in the Spirit. In various depictions of Christian saints, you'll see the Holy Spirit descending as a dove onto someone's shoulder or head and as a symbolic form depicting the Holy Spirit's presence in that individual and how it has transformed them into a saintly human being. The rite of baptism may be viewed as a ritual for passing on the grace of the Holy Spirit, another ritual form of giving shaktipat.

Kundalini isn't limited in any way. Shaktipat can happen in any state of consciousness—while you are awake or in dreams. You can meet a great master and have the experience of receiving a transmittal in a dream state; you can have a dream of a divine form—people have experiences of Shakti, of Kundalini, of the great Goddesses or Shiva, or other divine forms such as Buddha, Kwan Yin, and Tara. People have shared with me their experiences of Jesus coming and touching their forehead, and they got shaktipat. They had an awakening, and the transmittal of the Holy Spirit came through to them. In the yogic tradition, shaktipat is described as happening in a number of different ways. There can be specific rituals and practices that are designed to empower a person and transmit that power. But shaktipat can also happen spontaneously in a wide variety of situations. I mentioned many of these in the introduction— Kundalini can awaken in meditative or yoga practices, in prayer, in rituals, in intense martial arts training, in trauma, in near death experiences, during sex, while being with someone as they die, under the influence of drugs, and the list goes on and on. There are people who have experiences of awakening in dreams or visions where they are touched by a sage, a saint, Buddha, or some other enlightened being. People have told me of awakenings that occurred when energy suddenly surged in their body during very simple yoga practices, and they had a subsequent dramatic awakening experience.

In fact, in ancient yogic texts, there are numerous common circumstances that can lead to experiences of consciousness suddenly opening to what's beyond the ordinary mind. Awakening can even happen in a sneeze! A sneeze can still the mind, and in that stillness, there can be a flash of transcendent awareness in which one awakens to what lies beyond the confines of ordinary consciousness. This typically isn't Kundalini awakening, but when it happens that flash of transcendent awareness catches our attention and begins to make us wonder what we are really capable of experiencing. When Kundalini awakening does occur, through whatever means, it cuts through the root ignorance that binds our awareness to ego mind-body functioning.

There's a beautiful story that comes out of the ancient Vedic tradition that one of my early teachers told me. Before we're born, when we are in the womb, it is said that we repeat the mantra Shivo'ham, Shivo'ham, which means, "I am Shiva, I am Shiva. I am the absolute, I am the infinite." We swim in the blissful experience of our own Infinite nature. Then, as we go through the trauma of being born and pushed out into this world, we come out as a crying infant screaming, "Ko'ham, Ko'ham, Ko'ham," which means, "who am I, who am I, who am I," because in the agony of birth we've lost the experience of our Shiva nature, our infinite boundless nature. Then, from the moment we're born we are told, "You're a boy; you're going to be this. You're my son; I want you to become that. You're my daughter; you should be this. You're a girl, you can only do that." With covering after covering, limited identity after limited identity, we become a more limited form of who and what we are, and we're told that's who we are. We identify with it, we take it in, and we tell ourselves, "I'm a man, I'm a woman, I'm a husband, I'm a wife, I'm a son, I'm a daughter." All the things that come after "I am" become those coverings that limit and bind our consciousness to the small containers these identities provide.

It's shaktipat that cuts through all those coverings and begins to give us access to what our expanded infinite nature is and always has been. Those coverings don't have to be destroyed, we can fulfill our roles in the world, in our relationships; we can live in the world and not be bound by it. Some of these will be radically transformed because some of the containers, aspects of our limited ego mind, don't serve us very well. We still continue having the experience of our everyday life, but we are now informed by the knowledge and wisdom of what we truly are. With them come the boundless compassion, patience, and love that infuse our mind, life, and actions.

There are classic forms that shaktipat takes, which are described in the yogic literature. Shaktipat can come through the touch. Being touched by somebody who has awakened Kundalini, someone who has been empowered to convey Shakti, physically, through a touch will bestow shaktipat. Another form of shaktipat *diksha*, "initiation," can come through empowered mantra. Empowered mantra can serve as a vehicle for transmitting that extraordinary power of Consciousness.

In its highest form, mantra is a throb of the infinite power of Kundalini. Mantra is a primary means for conveying that power to another. All mantras, and in fact the entire Sanskrit alphabet, have their origin in Kundalini Shakti. When mantra comes through someone who has experienced and realized the power of that mantra, that mantra conveys the power to ignite the experience of true knowing within the mind and body of the recipient. Mantra is a classic and potent way of being able to pass on that power.

Thought is another means for giving shaktipat. The thought to give the blessing of shaktipat, arising in the purified mind of one who has been empowered by Kundalini to serve as her conduit, can transmit Kundalini Shakti to another person. In that sense, it is a thought of the Divine; it is a thought of the Infinite moving through the vehicle of the individual serving as a channel. It's the will of the Infinite, which is another form shaktipat can take, that passes through what we think of as thought, or we think of as mantra. But behind that is the power of Shakti, the will of Kundalini, and She uses these various forms as vehicles for conveying that power and igniting it within the individual. When I first met Swami Muktananda, I had no understanding, no idea that in that seemingly informal encounter, all the classic forms of conveying shaktipat were present. The ordinary mind simply doesn't know what is occurring on so many levels.

Shaktipat can even have occurred in a past life. People have told me of experiences, whether in a dream, or in a meditation, where they suddenly became aware that they received this initiation in a past life, and that's why it's continued to unfold in this life. That was my experience, in addition to receiving shaktipat many times in this life. One can always receive an influx of grace, of Shakti, even after Kundalini awakening.

I hear from people around the world who have had spontaneous experiences of Kundalini awakening. Most times they feel quite grace-full, and they're welcomed because of the awe and the beauty that they engender. Sometimes such awakenings can be scary or feel quite disruptive because the ordinary ego mind is going about its everyday life and suddenly it encounters movements (physical *kriyas*) in the body that may go with awakened Kundalini, or racing thoughts and feelings and visions and transpersonal experiences (subtle body kriyas) that the ordinary ego mind wasn't prepared for. Kriyas are movements of Kundalini impacting the mind and body. They are non-volitional, though they can be ameliorated. Integrating experiences of kriyas can be very challenging and there is guidance on this topic in chapter 14.

Kundalini is the boundless power of intelligence that is Universal Consciousness. She knows exactly what to give each seeker from awakening to completion, despite the ego mind's imposition of its judgment about whether or not the kriyas that go with the radical transformation are pleasant or unpleasant. This is something to watch out for. The ordinary ego mind steps back and judges your awakening and unfolding process, but Kundalini is what is unfolding. Kundalini changes your fundamental experience of who and what you are, what the nature of the universe is, and what all other beings in this universe are. It is only from that awareness that we go beyond the conditioned mind, beyond the ego, and beyond all of the mind's conditioned ways of reacting to everything in our environment and all the people we live with. By going beyond that conditioning, we are empowered by the radical freedom of our own infinite nature and its power of Consciousness, Kundalini.

KUNDALINI AS WITNESS CONSCIOUSNESS

Kundalini draws one into meditative states of Witness Consciousness. This is a shift in attention, a stepping back from the ordinary mind-body awareness and from the conventional sense of self that's defined by one's identification with it. It's a stepping back from all thoughts, all sensations, and all the things of the mind, and beginning to watch them from a place of clarity and freedom, with detachment and awareness, simply witnessing the flow of things through awareness. One may make use of mantra as a way that empowers our consciousness to be able to step back from its habit of identifying with everything going through the mind. Absorbing the mind in mantra disengages it from conditioned patterns of thinking and reacting. It's hard to simply step back from the mind that we've been identified with every waking moment of our lives. Every thought, every feeling has with it a sense of "that's me" and has with it a consciousness of "I'm that feeling, I'm that thought, I'm that person." In meditation, we begin stepping back and allowing ourselves to experience what it is to be free of the mind and all it produces.

Kundalini invites us to explore the expansive state of meditation, a state that goes beyond the ordinary states that we're familiar with: the waking state, the dream state, the deep sleep state. It invites us into an expanded state of awareness called *sahaja samadhi,* "living meditation," the state of Consciousness of Kundalini Shakti. We can become familiar with this state through the practice of bare awareness, Witness Consciousness, mantra, and through other practices (discussed in chapters 10 and 11) that allow the unfolding of infinite awareness, the unfolding of pure Consciousness, to inform our moment-by-moment experience.

One time in meditation, Shakti Kundalini said to me, "Be the seer, not the seen," and as I contemplated that, I became more and more aware of how whenever we're looking at something in meditation, we identify with it. A thought comes up in our mind, perhaps something we see, and we immediately identify with it in some way, we become what we see—whether what we're seeing is a thought, a feeling, the role that we're playing at that moment in life, or something else. "That's me, that's my thought, that's my feeling, that's what I'm doing," underlies all that we see, all that we perceive. But to step back and to keep stepping back, to simply be the Seer, the Witness, the one who sees but is never seen is what we're invited to know—that boundless awareness of simply Being, being the Seer, not the seen. That inner awareness is often referred to as Witness Consciousness, the ability to simply watch and see what arises in the mind, and what dissolves. You can do this right now.

> Watch what arises in the body and watch as the sensations and feelings dissolve. Simply watch whatever arises in the mind and watch as it dissolves in a matter of moments. Notice that there's a witness state of awareness that is unmoved by the movements of the mind, unmoved by the fluctuations and movements of the body.

That unmoving awareness, that unmoving state of the Witness, is what we can become more and more fully conscious of in each moment, whether in meditation or not. In time, it informs what we're doing in everyday life. The same process occurs in Buddhist practices such as mindfulness and *vipassana*—these are foundational practices for unfolding one's already awake and aware Buddha mind. When fully unfolded, the Witness is directly experienced as the Self, Shiva/Shakti.

Through practices that allow us to step back from the mind, we begin to see how the mind creates containers of awareness, containers of limited consciousness moment by moment. Each thought is a container and has associated with it some sense of identity—however fleeting it might be—it has some sense of "me" or "I" associated with it. Or it may be something like, "Oh, that's *not* me," in which case it is the dis-identification that equally defines us. These are constantly arising in the inner space of awareness. It is how the ego mind maintains its identity, constructing it moment by moment. The Witness is like the light that illumines that inner state; it illumines the inner sky of awareness, without judgment, without having to push anything away or hold it present, free of grasping, free of repulsion. The practice of entering into that Witness Consciousness where we can really step back and watch the mind can be done while you're doing daily tasks as well. In whatever your activity is, you can cultivate an awareness, a mindful state, where you're just watching with detached witness awareness.

Practicing Witness Consciousness makes us more and more aware of the patterns and influences that create our inner reality moment by moment. It gives us the detachment to see the big picture of our life as well, while watching from a place of equanimity as the winds and currents of emotions, thoughts, and desires sculpt our inner landscape. Witnessing allows us to become fully aware of what drives us forward in our life and why it drives us, empowering us to make more conscious choices about what we are cultivating and what we want to flourish.

WITNESS CONSCIOUSNESS MEDITATION

In this practice of Witness Consciousness as a meditation you set aside whatever you have to do in the moment, freeing your attention to really focus on that expansive, detached awareness, cultivating it and sustaining it for longer and longer periods—twenty, forty, or sixty minutes at a time.

Witness meditation practice empowers you to step back from the mind and body and is very steadying when kriyas are occurring, those movements of Kundalini that may physically impact the body or stir the mind in countless ways.

With each period of meditation practice, you strengthen your ability to detach from the habitual, compulsive identification with mind-body phenomenon and watch from the inner seat of equanimity, being the Seer not the seen.

The Seer is always present, even now as you read, the Seer watches the mind, watches the body, with boundless compassionate awareness. The Seer, the Witness, is the Self of all, Shiva, whose light of Consciousness is Shakti Kundalini.

To begin, find a comfortable posture for sitting. Sitting upright helps to support being awake and aware and alert, but if you have back problems or need to lie down, that's okay; it simply requires more vigilance to stay awake. What's most important is your posture of awareness, the posture of alertness, the posture of attentiveness that you're going to bring to this practice.

Sitting upright allows your breathing to be comfortably deep and full, which also supports being awake and aware, alert, giving your awareness the clarity to keep stepping back from the mind, but without going into the fogginess of sleep.

As you settle into a comfortable posture and you allow your awareness to begin to step back from the mind, start watching your breath. Just notice how the breath is coming in and going out. Feel the waves of the breath coming in and going out. Awareness just watches the flow of the breath, watching the waves of the breath. Invite the breath to slow and deepen.

Invite the breath to become more diaphragmatic, breathing from the tummy, more deeply and comfortably. Witness the feeling of the movement of the breath, feeling the air coming in and going out through your nose, at the same time feeling the rise and the fall of your abdomen. All the while, awareness just watches as a detached peaceful witness.

You may notice muscles soften and warm as they release and let go, while awareness remains clear and alert. Watching, just watching the movements of the body.

Watching the movements of the mind, awareness, like a clear light, illumines whatever arises in that inner sky of consciousness, the inner spaciousness of the mind.

Just watch whatever drifts by, a thought or a feeling, a memory or sensation—it doesn't matter. Like watching clouds drift by in a summer sky. The clouds can have different shapes and forms. And they don't move you or touch you in any way as you just watch them as the witness, detached and aware, relaxed and at ease, simply watching as though you're a bubble of awareness in this infinite expansiveness of space.

And you're watching that bubble as it breathes. Watching the breath flowing in, flowing out. Detached and aware. Spacious and free. Able to watch, watch the movements of the mind, the movements of the body. And just as things move through space, the space itself is unmoved—even if that movement is as grand as the movement of planets and stars, space remains untouched, unmoved.

In the same way, that spacious expansiveness of your awareness contains all the movements of the mind and body, but remains untouched, unmoved, steady—just watching—awake and aware. Keep watching until your timer goes off.

That steady awareness of the Witness resides within. That steady awareness is like an unwavering flame in a windless place. It radiates sublime, embracing, calming, loving awareness. That steady awareness resides within like a flame, a flame of awareness within the heart that can be seen in meditation. It is indescribably beautiful, and it radiates warmth, joy, clarity, and love. Once you've experienced it, you'll want to return to it over and over again. You can go back to that steady awareness, with its warmth and its love, its calming steady presence, over and over again, to take refuge in the heart, to take refuge in that awareness, to take refuge in the true nature of your own Self. Enjoy resting in your own Self more and more frequently, more and more fully, more and more permanently. This is the path to radical freedom.

6

The Soul's Yearning for Transcendence

Kundalini sadhana requires that we become aware of what drives us. What desires and yearnings are we consciously and unconsciously following? Many of our answers will create resistance to receiving Kundalini's inspirations and directions. Witness Consciousness helps differentiate the push and pull of the conditioned mind from Kundalini's currents moving you toward the Self. While practicing witness meditation, you may have been able to see more deeply into what you desire and what your soul yearns for.

Our culture is so steeped in psychology that most people's reflections on the source of their desires and yearnings, and why they have them, have a set of Western psychological assumptions that is part of the unconscious conditioned mind and how it views reality. These assumptions about what shapes our inner reality need to be made conscious. Family, peer groups, and culture are a few of the social-psychological factors that come to mind when we think about what influences how we learn what to value and what to desire, all of which drives us into a life of pursuing the fulfillment of those things with greater or lesser success. While wondering about where our desires and yearnings come from, we might also think of primary drives (thirst, hunger, sex, etc.) and secondary drives (wealth, power, status, etc.) that psychology delineates.

CONTEMPLATION

You may want to have your journal or notebook with you to jot down your wisdom as you do this exercise. Let your mind go back in time to when you were a teenager, perhaps in high school, and remember what that time was like as you prepared to move further out into the world of work or college, military service, or something else. What did you dream of becoming? What were you passionate about? Then as you grew older, how did your vision of yourself and what you would pursue in life change?

Education, work, careers, relationships, marriage, religious and spiritual pursuits can affect how we view ourselves as well as what our sense of purpose and meaning in life are. Did you feel called to do something?

Moving ahead in time to now, what do you most long for? What deep desires are in your heart? Allow these to come to awareness without any judgment, without any "shoulds" concerning what you should desire or yearn for.

You're giving yourself the open accepting space of awareness to allow the deepest parts of you to speak, to answer the questions: What do I truly want and need? What did I take birth for? What is the meaning and purpose of my life?

Some answers will arise quickly, while parts of yourself may be shy and need the patient openness of awareness to be coaxed into speaking their truth.

Gently repeat these questions to yourself one by one and see what arises each time you ask.

There's a quest in every question. Yours takes you deep within yourself and deep within your life.

The prize of wisdom, clarity, and insight is calling you.

Writing down what you discover is a way of valuing what you've been given from within. It will allow you to return to those discoveries to see how you are meeting those longings, how congruently you are living your profound sense of meaning and purpose in the moment, in this day, this week, in your relationships, in your work, and in relation to your highest nature.

Western psychology is great for giving us details about the formation and operation of the ordinary ego mind and how it develops normally or in maladaptive ways. It also provides us with useful information about neuropsychological and cognitive capabilities—emotions, stress, ordinary states of consciousness, life-span development, peak performance, and more. But traditional Western psychology doesn't offer much information about what lies beyond the ordinary mind. In fact, from the reductionist perspective of Western psychology, there is nothing beyond the material functioning of the body and brain. I'll go further into the differences between ancient yogic psychology and modern Western psychology in the next chapter.

The soul's yearning, our deepest and most soulful longing, may not make sense to many people. It may sound like a vague and elusive feeling. In Western psychology, our soul's yearning is considered to be merely a strong desire, without any deeper significance, because there is no such thing as the soul. There's just the firing of neurons and the conditioned responses of the organism, both cognitive and behavioral. We've forgotten that psychology originated as the study of the soul (psyche means "soul"). Early in the twentieth century, in its attempt to be scientific, Western psychology first lost its soul, and then it lost its mind, when even "mind" was deemed too unscientific to be studied!

As C. G. Jung, Joseph Campbell, and many other depth psychologists and mythologists showed, there are profound insights into our psychology revealed in dreams, visions, and myths, which is not where the dominant paradigm of cognitive-behavioral psychology typically looks for understanding human nature. Jung was the first Western psychiatrist with a model of psychological functioning that included a transcendent function. The Self in Jungian psychology is the psyche's transcendent function that serves to integrate all its aspects and also moves one toward higher levels of development and individuation. Jung saw evidence of this transcendent function operating in individuals and in groups through myths and symbols, dreams, religious ideologies. He also saw an innate drive for individuation, for higher levels of integration, creativity, and wisdom which incorporates information and energy from transindividual or transpersonal sources such as archetypal dreams, myths, and symbols.

Mythic journeys and mythic truths depicting transpersonal influences on the individual's development have been a part of human culture for tens of thousands of years. Mythic journeys and quests are symbolic representations of what individuals have been encountering on their journeys through life for millennia. They speak to the individual from a place of wisdom that transcends the personal, yet informs the individual by what can be seen of their journey from a higher level. Joseph Campbell has written about the structure of what he calls the *monomyth* of the hero's journey. Across countless reiterations, it conforms to one pattern regardless of whether one looks at the life of Jesus, Moses, or Buddha, Odysseus, the heroes of the Grail legend, the Pandavas in the Mahabharata, Milarepa, Mirabai, or thousands of other such figures. These are patterns that we can find in our own lives as each one of us is living the starring role in the hero's journey of our own creation. The transformative power of Kundalini can be understood as the power driving one forward on the greatest quest of all—the quest for wisdom, agapé, ecstasy, and the radical freedom of enlightenment.

PHASES OF THE HERO'S JOURNEY

Campbell discovered that the archetypal journey of the hero has three phases to it regardless of who the heroine or hero is, mythic or real. First, the journey demands that the hero leaves ordinary life in society—sometimes it's by choice; sometimes it's by circumstances or accidents that force them out of society and onto their quest. The hero or heroine is one who picks up the quest and is carried forward by transpersonal, archetypal, or mystical forces that are constellated by the quest. They summon what they can internally and externally to meet the demands of the quest, which, by its very nature, will require more than they will ever be able to gather alone. Secondly, the hero or heroine goes on a mythic journey during which they encounter supernatural forces or extraordinary situations that demand extraordinary responses from them and assistance from beyond the ordinary mind and everyday reality (may the force be with you!). In the process of meeting these demands, overcoming obstacles, persevering, discovering hidden supports, and so forth, they develop profound skills or strength, profound awareness, an open heart, deep compassion, or some other qualities. In this way they are initiated into a higher mode of being and functioning. As they reach the end of that segment of the hero's quest, after having been through the ordeal and initiation, they take possession of something of great value. It may be that they found it in some remote place or, in the archetype of the spiritual quest, it is found within. Lastly, the hero returns to their group or nation or humanity with the extraordinary prize to share it for the benefit of others. Campbell's book *Hero with a Thousand Faces* brilliantly discusses many examples of this archetypal journey.

Campbell summarizes the sequence of the hero's journey in three phases: leaving, initiation, and return. This sequence is repeated over and over again in countless myths. We even see it in modern myths. Joseph Campbell was a consultant on the original *Star Wars* trilogy. Luke Skywalker and what he went through depicted the myth of the hero's journey, as well as was his father's journey to the dark side and back. We see the hero's myth in what Frodo went through in *The Lord of the Rings* as well, and the list of movies and stories focusing on the hero's journey goes on and on: *Moses and the Ten Commandments, The Lion King, The Chronicles of Narnia, The Golden Compass, The Matrix* trilogy, the Harry Potter series, *Avatar,* and many others. The mythic journey is perennially engaging for people because it offers the deep wisdom necessary for understanding the profound meaning of a purpose-driven life. The higher the purpose, the greater the meaning, but also the greater the challenges and sacrifices demanded.

One of the greatest figures in modern history to have made the hero's journey is Mahatma Gandhi. Like most heroes, he began the quest without knowing it, unconscious of the powers within him and the transcendent powers around him that were driving him forward. His life began in 1869 in a conventional way within traditional Hindu culture. As was the custom then, he was married at age thirteen to a young Hindu girl who had been betrothed to him for years. He was an average student and an average athlete who had to work hard just to finish college. His father wanted him to study law in hopes of having him take over his position in government one day. Gandhi went to England to study law and returned to India afterward. His attempts to establish a successful law practice in India failed, in part because he was shy and couldn't effectively assert himself in court. Not long after the birth of his second child in 1892, he took a position as a lawyer in South Africa where the major turning point in his quest occurred.

The brutally racist, oppressive government and society of South Africa ignited his passionate pursuit of justice, equality, and freedom, while he remained steadfast to his absolute commitment to nonviolence, truth, simple living, and a love for God that transcended religious differences. Historically, the only way to bring about the massive changes in society and government that his ideals called him to seek was through violent upheaval and revolution. He completely rejected those paths and allowed the power of the principles of *ahimsa* (nonviolence), truth and justice, dharma, and his unflagging commitment to them to transform him and inspire him to create the way of nonviolent protest. He went from being an unimposing Hindu barrister, barely able to speak up in court, to a champion, a hero of freedom, justice, equality, and religious tolerance, able to move millions of people through the power of his words and his example. This didn't happen overnight. It didn't happen without titanic battles within himself and conflict with overwhelming powers of government and wealth that opposed him. But he heard the call and answered it. He persevered through vicious beatings and lengthy fasts, abstaining from food until he was at the brink of death more than once. Through it all, he remained true to his spiritual practices and beliefs, based on the ancient Vedas and the Bhagavad Gita, and overcame the greatest powers in the world.

In the process, he threw off many of the conventional beliefs and ways of his caste and culture. With humility, he simplified his life, rejecting materialism, as his political and spiritual power grew greater and greater. He became a *mahatma*, "a great soul." Like so many heroines and heroes, he not only lived in fulfillment of his quest, he sacrificed his life to it. On January 30, 1948, he was assassinated by a deeply afflicted religious zealot who opposed Gandhi's vision of Muslims and Hindus living in harmony with mutual respect. When Mahatma Gandhi was shot, all he uttered was, "Ram, Ram," the name of the Divine he had so steeped his heart and soul in; it was all there was to be revealed as his soul departed.

Gandhi's life led him through the stages of the quest. He wasn't thinking, "I'll go on a quest for freedom, justice, and equality and see what happens." Yet the archetypal pattern was there. Life events took him out of India into English culture and further cultivated the seeds of his ideals, which were already in him. When he returned to India, he failed to be successful in society at that time. The failure led him to South Africa and the confrontations that shaped his future path. The first phase of the journey is leaving behind one's conventional society. Phase two is the initiation. His was through the fire of the brutal beatings that he and his loved ones, friends, and followers endured. He discovered the transpersonal power of the principles he was adhering to. That transindividual power of truth and love transformed him. It transformed his ways of engaging others, confronting authorities, and gathering worldly power in the service of the highest. Having obtained the prizes of knowledge, wisdom, and power, he returned to India bringing these attainments into service of all humanity. His gifts continue to inspire and lead others on their quests for truth, justice, and equality.

MYTHIC JOURNEYS OF THE GODDESS

There are symbolic and mythic maps that offer guidance on how to traverse the metaphysical terrain of ego transformation for the soul's journey along the path of Kundalini. A great myth encapsulates layer upon layer of truth and wisdom that you can unfold as you study it and unravel the symbols that are speaking to you about your life journey. The mythic tale of the great goddess Kali communicates deep truths that are important to understand for Kundalini sadhana. Interestingly, Albert Einstein said that if you want your children to be intelligent, read them fairy tales, and if you want them to be really intelligent, read them *more* fairy tales.

There are mythic tales of the Goddess from other traditions that also convey deep wisdom applicable to Kundalini sadhana. There's an ancient story of the great goddess Inanna from thousands of years ago in the Sumerian civilization. The mythic tale of Inanna dates back to a time when the Goddess was honored and worshipped, though the patriarchal traditions were growing in power. Inanna was a great goddess, and there is a mythic tale of her descent into the underworld that required careful preparation. She had to pass through seven gates in her descent to the Great Goddess of the underworld, her sister Ereshkigal. At each gate, she is stripped of another part of her regalia, until she is finally totally naked, and forced into submission to confront the Goddess. It is a descent by choice, though it is terribly dangerous, and she ends up dead. But thanks to her preparation and the help of her divine uncle and two little insignificant beings he creates, she had her life restored by the goddess Ereshkigal. There's great wisdom in the details, too many to go into here, of her descent and the return ascent which brings Inanna great powers that she is able to use upon her return. On Kundalini's path, we are stripped of any attachment and identification with the personas we wear, the ways that the ego mind postures on the stage of its life. There's a symbolic death that happens in sadhana. Sylvia Brinton Perera wrote a brilliant book, *Descent to the Goddess*, that unfolds the deep wisdom of Inanna's tale.

Inanna's story is a mythic journey that is about a chosen descent. Inanna decided to go into the underworld as part of her hero's journey. In a later historical period, there's a myth that takes on a different inflection; it is the myth of Demeter and Persephone and Persephone's forced descent into the underworld. In this famous tale, the young goddess Persephone and her adoring mother, a mature goddess named Demeter (an earth goddess and wife of Zeus) are out in the countryside. Persephone is gathering flowers, when suddenly the earth splits open and out springs Pluto, Lord of the Underworld, brother of Zeus, who abducts her, dragging her into the underworld against her will. Demeter doesn't know what happened to her daughter; Persephone simply vanished. Demeter suffers tremendous grief and brings that grief to the entire world. Demeter was mourning the loss of her daughter, and as Goddess of the Earth, she withdrew her support of life on earth. Everything began to wither and die, all the warmth and life went out of the earth until she was finally able to recover her daughter, and then spring blossomed once again. There are many more details revealing important lessons for the soul about mourning, retrieving the parts of us lost in the underworld, betrayal and collusion, and more.

This mythic tale speaks to the times when our soul is captured and dragged into the underworld. Those are times when we haven't chosen to go on a hero's journey, but instead we're abducted; it may feel like the earth has suddenly opened up, and we fall into the abyss. This may be as a result of rape or abuse. The mythic tale is known as the Rape of Persephone. Hundreds of thousands of women, children, and men are suffering this horrific fate every year.

The feeling of abduction and forced descent may also happen when we've lost a loved one or our entire career has disappeared because of economic circumstances or disaster, accidents or death swallows everything. People who have suffered strokes, heart attacks, or severe injuries sometimes have the feeling of suddenly being abducted by illness, and their entire life changes for the worse, as if a hole opened up and swallowed their life. There's so much loss they experience.

We have thousands of military personnel coming back from areas of violent conflict transformed by the descent into the underworld of war, suffering trauma, injuries, and the death of friends and loved ones. It can be as if a fissure in the world opened up and swallowed their former life. This happened to people in the New York City area who survived the 9/11 attacks and lost loved ones in the attacks.

Persephone's story is a mythic tale of the Goddess that gives meaning and context for deepening our understanding of what happens in these forced descents. The human psyche has experienced these forced descents for all our existence. The mythic tales are the wisdom of our collective consciousness passed down through stories. They also help us to understand the great mythic quality that our life's journey has due to these kinds of dramatic and impactful events. We are living these great mythic dynamics that unfold in our life. We are not alone, and we aren't the first ones to traverse this terrain.

When we have the greater consciousness that comes with Kundalini awakening, it empowers us to step back and see the dynamics of this great and terrible drama unfolding; the hero's journey has no guarantee of a return in this life. Awakening empowers us to know we have within us the qualities that we can access and develop, the powers we need to come out of the underworld, to come back with some great gift, some great boon to pass on to humanity. Young, innocent Persephone masters the underworld and becomes Queen of the Underworld, with the power to go back and forth between worlds. Wounded soldiers discover their resiliency and power to overcome massive injuries and loss of limbs. Rape and abuse survivors discover how to move from victim to victor. These are the heroic journeys unfolding in people's lives all around us. The successful returns to fully living include the support of one like Demeter, the relentlessly supportive, ferociously loving mother who was not going to allow her daughter to remain trapped in the underworld. In a person's life, that figure might be an individual or a team, a therapist, a physician, loved ones, or other people who have suffered the same wounds and made it back.

These kinds of great myths give us a much broader, more expansive view of what our life is about, even when there are tragic circumstances that we have to deal with. Myths help us to understand what's needed to get through those circumstances successfully and what qualities, virtues, strengths, or wisdom we may be returning with that will benefit others. This mythic context helps us to understand what we are encountering on our soul's journey and what part Kundalini awakening plays in our mythic quest.

EVERYDAY HEROES ON THEIR JOURNEYS

Though we can see the same phases and dynamics of the hero's journey at play with other great historical figures, the truth is, I see them unfolding everyday in the lives of the people I encounter and the clients I work with. For some it is the dark journey of drugs and alcohol that makes them leave society and bottom out. Many of these people find their heroic journey brings them to surrender to a higher power and adherence one day at a time to the twelve-step structure that brings them wisdom, strength, and compassion. They return this to others in need of the same healing power. I see people on their quests reclaiming the power to love and be loved after having grown up abused and neglected. There are countless heroic journeys of people serving in the armed forces, the Coast Guard, in police and fire departments, as first responders, nurses, physicians, parents, caretakers of loved ones, and on and on. Every walk of life has quiet heroes walking the archetypal transpersonal path through their dedication to the ideals and values that take them beyond themselves. Your heroic journey is your very next step, your very next breath. You don't have to be some grand figure. In fact, humility is one of the most valuable virtues summoned by the quest.

On the archetypal journey of awakened Kundalini, one becomes more and more empowered to view one's life and the dynamics of it from a transcendent and transpersonal perspective. One of Kundalini's expressions is the intensified yearning to be free, to go beyond all that is familiar. The intent of Kundalini is to empower us to look beyond the details of our individual life and see the greater dynamic process. In so doing, we're in the phase of the hero's journey of stepping outside of the ordinary dynamics of family, friends, and culture, transcending them so that we can extricate our consciousness from them, as well as gain the power to act more skillfully within them.

Kundalini unfolding, the path to radical freedom, is the soul's journey; it is the great archetypal quest, the nivritti phase of cessation, of freeing oneself from forms, from malas, and the conditioned ego mind. It involves heroic encounters right in the context of your life as it is. It is a journey to the Infinite without going anywhere. It is a journey of absolute transcendence while becoming fully alive and present in your life now. It answers your deepest yearnings for freedom, purpose, meaning, and love.

In our materialist culture, the purpose and meaning of life are often defined by career goals, financial ambitions, status, wealth, possessions, and physical appearance. The notion that one's quest for purpose and meaning will be fulfilled through career success, financial rewards, and so forth, is itself a myth, but it's the prevailing myth so it often becomes unconscious, unquestioned, and taken for granted that the acquisition of these things *should* drive us. However, it is a myth that leaves people spiritually starved. In that myth we're primarily driven by desires for survival, possessions, sex, and power—interestingly, all functions of just the first three chakras! The ordinary ego mind is consumed by fulfilling these drives, and Western psychology offers guidance on many of the dynamics related to fulfilling those desires in socially acceptable ways. Jung remarked once that if someone shows signs of the fourth chakra, the heart chakra, they might be called a saint, so rare is this higher influence! Of course from a yogic perspective, there's a great deal more to the journey beyond the fourth chakra.

Kundalini awakening is often challenging for people because it re-awakens the questioning of prevailing cultural myths and values that have been part of what shaped their entire lives. This is the phase of stepping outside of society on your quest, leaving it behind in certain ways. We live in a massive group that shapes the development of the mind from the moment we're born. When we think of a cult, we often think of a group that brainwashes people, limiting members' thinking in severe ways. But we forget that we all live in a cult-ure. We grow up and develop as a member of a group that confines our thinking and restricts our freedom, whether it's through culturally defined roles of a man or a woman or a race, or whether it's where we stand in society or our family or religion—all of these impose limitations on the mind. The processes of awakening and unfolding Kundalini challenge us to get free of those patterns of conditioning, to step outside of them and reclaim our radical freedom. Only then are we empowered to consciously choose the patterns that can serve the expression of our highest nature.

Some of the people I work with are very successful professionals, entrepreneurs, investors, and business people who encounter the clash between their awakened consciousness and how it contrasts with the suddenly old lifestyle, values of friends, family, business peers, and the culture they live in. It can feel very isolating. Instead of feeling tremendously successful due to their money, power, and accomplishments, they may go through a period of feeling trapped by them and by the limited identity associated with them. They then need support for learning how to get through the feelings of soul suffocation without simply abandoning their lives in search of a freedom that must be found within.

Wealth and worldly success are not inherently opposed to spiritual growth, but being driven by lack and want is. The striving of such individuals is typically compelled by ambition, possessiveness, and cravings for power, money, and pleasure, binding one to a state of deficiency and limitation that clashes with Kundalini's one-pointed drive to free everyone from the conditioned ego mind.

Awakening, becoming conscious of all this, can throw people into deep soul-searching, reevaluating what they truly cherish and believe, and gradually separating their genuine Self from the false self of the conditioned mind, discerning the difference between their Infinite nature and their conventional self. Once the mind is transformed, an individual will make use of all their karmas and resources—including wealth, power, or fame—to act selflessly in accord with their innate qualities of boundless compassion, kindness, generosity, and love.

THE CHALLENGE TO TRANSCEND AND INCLUDE

Our awakened consciousness makes us look at the things that bind us, the things that restrict us, the ropes of beliefs and assumptions that our mind has to climb out of and leave behind like the butterfly emerging from its chrysalis. Kundalini shines the light of Consciousness on the beliefs that shape our experiences, what we should pursue, what we should avoid, what relationships should be like, our fears and our longings. Kundalini confronts us with these elements of the conditioned mind and how actions in the moment reveal the limitations of ego—in interactions with our family, friends, coworkers, teachers, while waiting in line at a grocery store or driving in traffic. Kundalini, one's own power of Consciousness, is unlimited in her ability to use any and all situations to teach us and guide us to freedom. Kundalini is the inner master teacher, the inner power of revelation and transformation, for whom there is no time, no place, no state in which the ego, the limiting and binding self-sense, can hide. She's always present performing her sacred task of delivering you from ignorance and suffering if you choose to listen. *She loves you as her very Self and wants you to know the full delight of being who you truly are.* She is the soul's yearning for radical freedom and transcendence.

Through C. G. Jung's work, Western psychology became informed of the transcendent function, the Self, and its role in developing higher order integration, even if it was never embraced by mainstream psychology. Yoga psychology has looked at human development from the transcendent perspective of the Self for thousands of years. It recognizes that we have an innate drive to transcend, to go beyond the ordinary limits of the body and ego mind. There are countless mundane expressions of urge to go beyond: some people push beyond human limits in artistic expression, others engage in intense sports performance, some feel driven to break the speed of sound on land or in the air. Science is very often pushing into new frontiers. Adventurers and explorers travel from the depths of the ocean to the highest mountaintops and outer space. Humans are constantly striving to transcend in order to experience greater freedom, power, knowledge, and joy. Beneath this seeking, we can see the five powers (to create, to sustain, to destroy, to conceal, and to reveal) of our Infinite Self operating in diminished forms, seeking release from the primal delusion of limited selfhood that produce the contracted state of the ordinary mind. Kundalini, the power of revelation and transformation, grants release from that bondage. Buddha exemplifies what it is to go beyond the conditioned mind, beyond all cravings, to live in unimaginable freedom. He became known as a tathagata, one who has gone beyond. He returned from his quest and gave a way to freedom accessible to all humanity, modeling boundless compassion as integral to freedom.

Relationships are another common way that people seek the joy of transcendence by attempting to lose their self in another person and in the experience of passionate love, dissolving the confines of ego boundaries in merging. This is why spiritual writings so often resort to analogies of love, union, and passion when attempting to convey the mysteries of dissolving into the Divine. Merger in human relationships is a limited form of transcendence that can delude people, giving a false sense of expansion and wholeness. Because of this, it can lead to codependence and addictive behaviors in relationships. In healthy relationships, loving union is an expression of each person's wholeness and supports them on their journey of exploring the Infinitude of their own being.

As I pointed out in chapter 4, the chakra system gives a map of how transcendence unfolds on the path of Kundalini and is meant to develop inclusively. Transcendence and inclusion are what produce higher orders of integration. Transcendence alone produces unconscious splitting and leaves areas of the ego mind untransformed. It's very hard work to transcend and include, transcend and subsume, transform and integrate all the levels from the bound ego mind struggling to exist, all the way up to the most expansive and radically free domain of the Infinite. It's much easier to find ways to experience transcendence and then attempt to abandon or denigrate what was left behind. But those unintegrated, untransformed parts continue to operate and eventually bring pain and suffering. This is especially evident in false teachers who have had genuine transcendent experiences but didn't complete the transformative and integrative work on all levels. I highly recommend reading Ken Wilber's comprehensive work on mapping out human experience and the importance of transcendence and inclusion. His book *Integral Psychology* has a valuable overview.

In sadhana, dedicated spiritual practice, we have to combine the yearning for freedom and transcendence with discrimination in order to discern whether we're being drawn by the ordinary mind's attraction and aversion patterns or powered by Kundalini to transform, transcend, and include what we're confronting. The ego mind can't do this alone; it can't jump out of its own way. Trusted teachers and fellow seekers can give the feedback the ego mind needs to truly see what pattern is unfolding in the moment. The ego mind often resists acknowledging the fabric of interdependence within which it exists. It intuits the source of wisdom and freedom within and would like to race there on its own, as if there were such a thing as its separate existence; its aloneness, its self-sufficiency, its rugged individualism are simply part of the delusion that the ego mind lives in. We are all interconnected and completely interdependent, indivisible on the most profound levels. We wouldn't even find a path, much less take steps along it, without the help of countless others who are here now and from those wise ones who have traversed the way in the past, generously leaving behind markers and directions.

We bring our wounded, afflicted, deluded mind (of which our ego is often so proud!) to our quest, to Kundalini unfolding, and may confront unhealthy merging and false transcendence in relation to spiritual groups, teachers, or other practitioners. There's no shame in that. It's simply another set of ego dynamics that needs to be seen and worked with skillfully, which may include psychotherapy. You are not your mind; you are not the patterns and habits of your mind that make up a conventional sense of self. You can look at the mind/self with clarity and compassion, free of defensiveness, and use all the resources that are available to reshape the mind. Supported by Kundalini, you are creating a new container, a new vessel for Consciousness to inhabit. Create it with great love and respect, great care, fashioning it in ways that will allow it to serve with joy as your journey unfolds. We learn to do this from models of greater consciousness, compassion, and integration that we find in teachers and fellow seekers. Having the humility to learn is one of the requirements of the path.

MOKSHA: LIBERATION AND TRUE FREEDOM

The journey on which Kundalini sadhana takes you leads to true freedom. In the yogic traditions, *moksha,* or liberation, is attained as the fulfillment of one of the great purposes of life. It is attained by living in the truth of who you are. There are irreducible qualities of your essential nature: boundless consciousness, boundless love, boundless compassion, boundless patience, and boundless joy. When we talk about radical freedom, it's the freedom to know these qualities and to be able to effortlessly live them at all times and in all places. Too often, we are barely able to muster enough patience, kindness, and compassion for our most deeply loved family members. We lose our patience with them. We lose our patience with ourselves. People lose their patience even with their own helpless infants, slapping them verbally or physically, even shaking them to death in frustration. If a person does that with loved ones, what happens with acquaintances? What happens with strangers? What happens with enemies?

The conditioning of the ordinary mind prevents us from being able to act with the radical freedom needed to express our true nature in any and all encounters with all other beings. The unfolding of our freedom is the unfolding of the qualities of compassion, love, generosity, and patience. Kundalini sadhana offers a path for clearing away the obstacles blocking us from both knowing the Self in the moment and being able to act effortlessly on those highest qualities of our Buddha nature, Christ consciousness, or Self. This is what the soul yearns for when it has matured and is ripe for awakening. Not every soul is at that stage. They may have many lifetimes to go before awakening is possible.

For some years in the late 1970s and early '80s, I volunteered to do weekly meditation programs in prisons for inmates, simply bringing basic practices into that kind of context to help individuals. It was a very profound experience for me, because if you think of a context where people are most suffering and most bound, prison has to be it, especially if you've seen it from the inside. In these programs, I would often do the simple foundational practices, as they are so powerful and absolutely essential. One inmate in particular stands out in my mind.

He had been referred because of his uncontrolled high blood pressure. It was suggested to him that he come to the weekly meditation program that I was leading. Many people come to meditative practices for health reasons such as stress, high blood pressure, anxiety, and many more, but the benefits go far beyond these as this inmate would discover.

He was serving a life sentence without parole for murder. When he came, he was very quiet, virtually never speaking, but week after week I saw through his body language how he was relaxing, how he was changing. After about two or three months of coming, just eight to twelve sessions, the clinical psychologist who had referred him got in touch with me and said, "You know, he was referred to you because he had uncontrolled hypertension. Now his blood pressure is not only under control, it's under control without medication; he was even able to go off medication. He's had a really amazing turnaround in his health."

The inmate continued to attend. Barely speaking, he'd come in, and we would do practices that included simple hatha yoga stretches, chanting the mantra Om Namah Shivaya, meditation on the detached witness awareness, and mantra meditation. Om Namah Shivaya means, "I honor the Auspicious One, the Divine within." But more importantly that ancient mantra comes from a source that is alive with the power to awaken a person's Kundalini, unfolding the awareness of who and what they are beyond the mind. Baba Muktananda told me to give people the mantra Om Namah Shivaya through which they could receive shaktipat.

Four or five months after this inmate began coming to the programs, he came up to me one night at the end of the session and told me he was about to be transferred to another prison. He said, "I have to tell you something. You know, I've been coming here, and my life has completely changed." He went on to say, "My whole life I've been told what a horrible ____ I am" and he used every four-letter word you might imagine, because he'd been called those things by his family, by the guards, by everyone. It turned out the man was thirty-four years old, and he had already spent seventeen years in prison. He told me he would never get out. He said, "Now, you came in here and you told me that there's something about me that's divine." He said, "I've never heard that in my life." He said, "But you didn't just tell me that, you gave me a way to try to really know that. You gave me this mantra and meditation practices. I just did what you told me; I started just silently repeating Om Namah Shivaya to myself."

He then began describing experiences that he was having in his prison cell, in a federal penitentiary, serving life without parole. They were the experiences of being visited by the Divine and being embraced by love, being embraced by light, being immersed in sounds that were unimaginable and unknown to him. So much so, that "In the end," he said, "even though I'll be in prison for the rest of my life, I'm freer now than I have ever been." He said, "The guards are going to continue to tell me what a horrible person I am. I'm going to have to live all my life in prison—and I deserve to," he said, "but I never have to believe what they tell me about who I am anymore, because now I know."

That freedom, regardless of what one's life is like, is what every one of us has available to us; it's what we yearn for. If an inmate in a penitentiary serving a life sentence can gain access to that, which one of us can't? Which one of us can't bring that freedom and that deep knowing into our everyday life? Can there be any excuse for not seizing the precious opportunity of a human birth to know the highest and pass it on? The highest knowing is the gift of Kundalini awakening. That's the turning point in the soul's journey that empowers Consciousness to transcend and include one's everyday life, informed as it is by the direct experience of Divine Love and Unity Consciousness. This inmate said, "Now my cell isn't a prison cell, now my cell is a monk's cell, and now my cell is a place for connecting with the Divine." That kind of transformation is a transformation of body and mind, it's a transformation of character, and it's a transformation of consciousness. These are the kinds of transformations that Kundalini produces in re-creating the mind and body so they can live in that extraordinary state. One's yearning for true freedom is fulfilled by Kundalini's gifts of grace.

The process of Kundalini awakening is the process of deepening your access to the Source, the source of your strength, your creativity, your powers, your wisdom, your internal source; your freedom is truly yours.

7

Yoga Psychology and Western Psychology

The ancient psychology of yoga offers many insights into how the mind and consciousness function—and many of these insights are in direct contrast with Western psychology's paradigm on how the mind and consciousness work. Our culture is steeped in psychology, to such an extent that most people aren't aware of it. For example, at another time or in another culture, if someone were behaving badly or strangely, their actions would have been explained by influences from the stars or the planets, or blamed on demons or possession; in some cultures it would have been attributed to spells and witchcraft. In our culture, if somebody is acting strangely or in a way that seems abnormal, we'll speculate about painful childhood experiences, upbringing, and family influences, or what they've been rewarded for and learned from peer groups. We might even wonder whether a disease or a tumor of the brain would cause such behavior. Our explanations are psychological and medical. They are very useful as far as they go, and that's why they are the dominant paradigm. We operate from a Western psychological paradigm, barely aware of its implications. For this reason, it's important to take a moment to look at a few of the basic assumptions of traditional Western psychology.

These are assumptions that many of us hold without being aware of them or without having consciously examined them recently. They are assumptions and beliefs about how our mind and consciousness operate that may clash with those of yoga and other Eastern and Western spiritual traditions. When different paradigms come into contact, such as our implicit Western psychological one and a spiritual or yogic one, there can be a clash that results in misperceptions and misunderstandings. Understanding one's own paradigm and the assumptions of the other paradigm can help reduce the misperceptions and miscommunications between the two.

Thomas Samuel Kuhn, physicist, historian, and philosopher of science, famously wrote about paradigm clashes in the history of scientific development. A paradigm includes the system of beliefs, concepts, values, and techniques of investigation that dominate the thinking of a community—scientific, yogic, religious, or other—during a given period in its history.[1] Over time, the basic assumptions of the dominant paradigm become implicit and unconsciously order one's thinking, perception, and theories of the nature of reality. For example, who thinks of gravity as a theory that may be false? Due to the successful nature of the theoretical constructs of gravity, they are taken for granted to be "real" and not just theory. We still don't know what gives mass gravity or where the force of gravity comes from.

Kuhn demonstrated that in the history of science, bringing together two disparate paradigms for comparative study or integration often results in "paradigm clash." The implicit, unrecognized basic assumptions of the dominant paradigm lead to incorrect deductions and conclusions when examining the competing paradigm. Eastern, yogic, and transpersonal paradigms on the one hand, and traditional Western psychological paradigms on the other, are in such a clash.[2] Unless the underlying assumptions of each system are understood and taken into account during any comparisons, paradigm clash and resultant distortions or false evaluations ensue.

Traditional Western psychology refers primarily to the cognitive-behavioral and psychoanalytic schools of psychology. It is in contrast to those schools of thought that yoga psychology differs the most. Two other prominent schools of psychology are humanistic and transpersonal psychology. Yoga psychology is more similar to them and nearly indistinguishable from transpersonal psychology on the level of basic assumptions. By yoga psychology, I mean the system codified by Patanjali (the great sage and codifier of yoga approximately two thousand years ago) and applied through the non-dualistic schools of Advaita Vedanta and Kashmir Shaivism.

If we compare a larger more inclusive paradigm with a smaller more restricted paradigm, misunderstandings and erroneous conclusions occur. The multiple states of consciousness model, held by meditation disciplines or consciousness disciplines, including yoga and other traditions of meditation or prayer, is considerably broader than the traditional Western psychological one in its view of the range of functioning of human consciousness. Thus, when the Western model is applied to Kundalini, yoga, or the consciousness disciplines, these Eastern psycho-spiritual systems and the qualities of consciousness they describe may be viewed as pathological or nonsensical and simply labeled or dismissed as unreal.

I had a Freudian psychology professor in graduate school who became apoplectic at my mentioning higher states of consciousness and out-of-body, near-death, or past-life experiences because in his view all such experiences were invalid and pathological. From his perspective, consciousness was a function of biological processes, unable to exist apart from the body and ceasing with death. This is what happens when the smaller more restrictive model, in this case psychoanalytic psychology, is applied to phenomenon included in the larger model. From the perspective of yoga psychology, the traditional Western paradigm is a useful model within its limits, but mustn't be misapplied to states of consciousness outside its scope.

Traditional Western psychology is in an analogous relationship to the consciousness disciplines as Newtonian physics is to Einsteinian physics: it is a subset of the broader, more inclusive model. Transpersonal psychology is a paradigm that attempts to encompass and integrate the entire range of human functioning, from the most sublime states considered by the consciousness disciplines to the most restricted pathological states delineated by traditional Western psychology. Ken Wilber's writings are among the best for understanding the transpersonal psychology model.

Four central points highlight the differences in the basic assumptions of the paradigms of the yogic or consciousness disciplines and traditional Western psychology:

1. Whether or not our normal, waking state of consciousness is optimal or suboptimal.
2. Whether or not true higher states of consciousness exist.

3. Whether or not higher states of consciousness are attainable through training.

4. Whether or not verbal communication is adequate for the communication of knowledge, especially the knowledge gained from higher states of consciousness.[3]

The consciousness disciplines hold that the waking state is suboptimal, that higher states of consciousness exist and are attainable, and that verbal communication about them is limited. Traditional Western psychology holds an opposing position: the waking state is the optimal state of consciousness; other states are suboptimal, irrelevant, or pathological; and intellectual analysis based on verbal encoding of experience is the highest form of knowledge.[4]

Traditional Western psychology reflects the materialistic philosophical position characteristic of the physical sciences prior to the impact of quantum physics. The materialist perspective is particularly evident in Freudian and cognitive-behavioral psychology. Both look to the material, the biophysiological, to explain the nature of human beings. Even Freud, who brought to the fore the powerful impact the unconscious has on the conscious mind, was a materialist, writing: "All our provisional ideas in psychology will someday be based on an organic substructure."[5] There are many psychiatrists, neurologists, neuropsychologists, and psychologists who believe we're virtually at that point now. They think they can write about Buddha's brain and accurately describe what his consciousness is like based on brain function, thus dismissing any existence of previous incarnations or the development of consciousness across lifetimes. Materialist science assumes that who we are is limited to and defined by our physical body and brain. A materialist scientist is always going to seek to reduce consciousness and Kundalini to physical events and processes. People speculate about Kundalini being caused by photon emissions and other physical phenomena. This only reflects the limitations of material science and the reductionism of scientific researchers. From the perspective of the yogic and meditative disciplines, Consciousness exists free of the material brain. This is a major clash point.

Traditional Western psychology seeks to explain the subtle in terms of the gross, assuming that the gross, physical level of reality (physiology, brain chemistry, sensory functioning, etc.) causes the subtler phenomena of consciousness (awareness, Consciousness, intuitions, etc.). Thus, the range of valid human experience is limited in such psychologies to those related to material existence. Altered states of consciousness, mystical states of union and ecstasy, trans-body or out-of-body experiences, post-death experiences, and other forms of transpersonal experiences are dismissed by traditional Western psychology as pathological, regressive, or merely subjective. At times, the behaviorists have either ignored or denied the existence of consciousness, viewing it as a mere epiphenomenon of biological functioning. The newer Western psychologies, humanistic and transpersonal, have been greatly influenced by yoga psychology and integrate Eastern psychological concepts into their frameworks.

YOGA VERSUS WESTERN PSYCHOLOGY: BASIC ASSUMPTIONS

Yoga differs from Western psychology in its assumptions about

1. the nature of the universe.
2. the nature of consciousness,
3. the nature of a human being,
4. the levels of functioning of the human mind,
5. the foundations of human suffering, and
6. how relief from suffering is gained.

You might find it interesting to take a moment and reflect on your ideas and beliefs concerning these six areas.

From the yogic perspective, there is only one "stuff" of this universe, and that is pure unbounded Consciousness, what we might call the Infinite Spirit of God, or Shakti. It is therefore monistic, not simply monotheistic. In the yogic tradition *pure* means untainted by any limiting form and untainted by any duality, in other words: no pairs of opposites, no subject-object split, no self and other; all there is, is the Self of All—God, Shiva, Shakti, the One. Yoga asserts that pure Consciousness contracts to become the universe nearly like the physicists' notion of energy taking the form of matter. The nature of the universe is Consciousness; every wave, every particle is a manifestation of Consciousness. Thus, it is the subtle that creates the gross, Consciousness that creates the body and exists independently of the body.[6]

Yoga psychology views healthy human functioning as inclusive of various states of consciousness and experiences that transcend body awareness. Like many spiritual disciplines, it prescribes specific methods for bringing about experiences of who we are beyond our body and our mind. For traditional Western psychology, consciousness can't exist independently of the body, since consciousness is assumed to be materially caused and biologically based.

Yoga holds that:

1. The nature of the universe is that of pure Consciousness manifesting in various forms or levels of contraction.

2. The nature of pure Consciousness, though beyond words, is described as eternal, boundless Being, Consciousness, and Bliss. When Consciousness identifies with a limiting form, it reflects the attributes of that form, whether it is inanimate, vegetative, animal, human, or transcendent.

3. The essential nature of a human being is pure Consciousness, the nameless Infinite, which bears many names.

4. The mind functions on a variety of levels broadly described by the three states of consciousness recognized by Western psychology (waking, dreaming, and deep sleep) and a fourth, recognized by yoga: the unlimited state of the Self called the *turiya* state.

5. The foundation of human suffering is twofold: the relative cause of suffering and the absolute cause. The relative cause is the lack of certain basic needs such as food, shelter, warmth, and so on. Western psychology also holds this view. The absolute cause of suffering is ignorance of the Self, wrong identification, and considering our self to be the mind-body complex rather than the Self of All, the Infinite, or Buddha mind.

6. Yoga focuses on the absolute cause of suffering, which is relieved only by direct knowledge of our true identity with the Divine. All of yoga is aimed at bringing about the recognition and experience of our true essential nature as pure unbounded Consciousness.

Indeed, working toward Self-realization is viewed as the highest human endeavor and the specific aim of all yoga disciplines. Yoga psychology envisions us becoming as established in the fullness and completeness of our highest Self as we are currently established in the limited and wanting nature of our bound self. How different this is from Freud's vision of successful psychotherapy as "changing the extreme suffering of the neurotic into the normal misery of human existence."[7] Western psychology is in the early stages of developing cognitive-behavioral approaches to positive psychology and health psychology, though they remain materialist in their basic assumptions.

Yoga psychology recognizes the three common states of consciousness and a fourth state, the turiya state of super-consciousness, or Self awareness. Compared to the turiya state, the waking state is severely limited, if not a state of delusion. Turiya is the ever-present, pure I-consciousness of the Self, Witness of the three usual states of consciousness. It is the ultimate state of Consciousness, the rapturous state of perfect unity awareness described by mystics of all traditions. Turiya is the state that subsumes the other three states, illuminating them with Consciousness. Turiya consciousness is experienced by adepts as eternal, uncaused, omniscient, and omnipresent. It is indistinguishable from the Self. The real nature of the turiya state is unutterable, unapproachable by speech, words, or the ordinary mind.

Typically we experience only an infinitesimal fragment of turiya in the form of a continuous sense of I-ness that persists through all the discontinuity of the various states of mind and consciousness comprising reality. We may intuit that there is something greater about ourselves than we already know, but the true vastness, the infinite expanse of our I-ness, our Selfhood, is beyond the reach of our imagination. *Attempting to know the Self with the mind is like trying to illumine the sun with a broken piece of a mirror.* It is the Self's irreducible quality of Consciousness that enables the Self to be the illuminating source behind the mind, the senses, and the body. From the perspective of yoga psychology, knowing the pure "I" in its fullness is the highest aim and purpose of human evolution.

Eastern disciplines and yoga psychology in particular assert that the highest state and the direct experiential knowledge of turiya are beyond the mind and words. To get to it, one must leave behind the mind and rationality. This assertion is in sharp contrast to the basic assumptions of traditional Western psychology, which views reasoning as the highest skill and the written word as the least ambiguous, most accurate way of transmitting our greatest knowledge. Mystics of every tradition become mute when asked to describe union with the Absolute, or resort to poetry and symbols that point beyond themselves.

Over the course of thousands of years, yogis have studied the various states of consciousness available to humans and concluded that our normal waking state is primarily one of delusion similar to the dream state. They come to this conclusion from the vantage point of what yoga psychology considers to be the highest state of consciousness, the turiya state mentioned earlier. From this perspective the other three states of consciousness are Self-imposed limitations and negation of Infinite Consciousness.

STATES OF CONSCIOUSNESS CONDENSING

Yoga psychology maps out in a variety of ways how the process of limiting pure transcendent Consciousness results in the restricted state of consciousness we are familiar with. One map looks at three phases of this process. These three stages correspond with the three ordinary states of consciousness—deep sleep, dreaming, and waking. I touched on these briefly in the previous chapter.

The deep sleep state is the state of the causal body; it is the awareness of no-thingness. It comes about by negation of the true all-encompassing state of Consciousness of the Self through the Self's power of concealment, Maya Shakti. This Self-negation, as noted earlier, is called avidya (primal ignorance). It's the beginning of the notion of limited individuality, the ego sense, and identification with limitations. Thus, instead of experiencing oneself as universal and unbounded, one thinks of oneself as a limited individual. It's the negation of one's true nature, the denial of one's true Self, and the identification with a limited part of that Self. It's referred to as the causal body due to the fact that this negation of, or dis-identification from, one's true nature, causes all that follows. This is the root cause of the contraction of Consciousness into the limited forms of mind and body as we know them. They evolve from that initial negation of universality. It is the root of all suffering.

In the deep sleep state there's only the awareness of nothingness. The Universal Self has been negated or dis-identified with so we're not conscious of that, yet the world of particulars, and the thoughts, desires, and details of individual existence, have not yet arisen. This state can be clearly experienced in meditation, illuminated by Kundalini Shakti. We experience it in deep sleep, but as we are dissociated from our fully conscious witnessing Self, the experience of that state is the black void of deep sleep. We know we had a deep sleep, we know we spent some time being aware of nothingness, but we never stop to think how that could be. This is a classic Vedantic argument demonstrating the presence of the Self as the Conscious Witness of the mind's various states.[8]

How can we be aware of being aware of nothingness? What part of us remains conscious even in deep sleep when we're not aware of the world, our body, or our mind? Who is the one who is conscious as we dream and reports the dream to ourselves? From the yogic perspective, it's the ever-present, ever-conscious Witness that is our Self, and we can never be truly separated from it, no more than the wave can be divided from the ocean. Our suffering and our quest arise only from our being unconscious of our unity with it. Even in deep sleep the Self is accessible. The ever-present illuminating Consciousness of the Self allows us to experience the nothingness of deep sleep as well as the contents of the other states of consciousness. If we shift our awareness to the Witness, the Experiencer of that state, then we can know our union once again.

From the causal body arise the subtle body and the physical body with their attendant states of dreaming and waking. The subtle body experience is basically the mind, thoughts, emotions, attitudes, and so on. It's the subtle sense of "I" compared with the gross sense of "I" associated with the physical body. The dream state reflects our identification with the mind and the subtle senses of which it is comprised. The subtle body isn't bound by the physical laws governing the physical body; thus, the experiences and actions of the subtle body during dreams seem nearly incomprehensible to the mind identified with the physical body in the waking state. However, while in the subtle body, one can have experiences that seem "paranormal," out-of-body, or post-death. During the course of yogic practices, such experiences may occur, especially in meditation through awakened Kundalini, and are taken to indicate the expansion of one's awareness beyond the confines of one's physical body.

Yoga psychology describes the mind and its workings in great detail. In some ways, it is similar to the various descriptions of the mind and personality developed by Western psychology. For example, yoga psychology includes concepts of ego, the unconscious, and processes of projection, identification, and conditioning. However, the origin and context are quite dissimilar. Three of the most salient features of the context in which the mind is viewed in yoga are its relation to bondage and liberation, its existence over time, and the condition of the mind in various states of consciousness.

Yoga views the mind as the cause of bondage and liberation. It creates bondage by thinking it is not the Self and that it is this particular, limited individual. Universal Consciousness becomes bound to individual consciousness.

That negation of infinite wholeness creates an identity that is wanting and incomplete. Yoga asserts that the mind then creates the senses, the body and the physical world to roam in, searching for wholeness, completeness, a total identity. The Self, that which is omnipotent, seems powerless and seeks to gain power, perhaps by pumping iron or by scaling the corporate ladder. That which is omniscient seems unknowing and seeks to raise its consciousness through therapy, growth groups, Eastern disciplines, and courses. That which is eternal seems bound in time and seeks to avoid death and leave a legacy by which to be remembered. The eleventh-century sage Kshemaraja, commenting on the Shiva Sutra, Limited knowledge is bondage (III:2), explains:

> Limited knowledge of the embodied individual becomes the cause
> of bondage. Firstly, in practical life we have to do with particulars.
> Therefore, the empirical individual thinks that particulars are the sole
> truth of life. He is confined to the differences and distinctions and is
> unable to grasp the Universal of which the particulars are only a limited
> expression. . . .
> Secondly, all the ideas of the individual are derived from sensori-
> motor perceptions, their images, and thought-constructs, imagination
> and fancies of the mind. . . . He is unable to believe that there can be
> a supersensuous reality. So he builds a prison for himself in which he
> takes the utmost delight to live.
> Thirdly, he considers his mind-body complex, his psychophysical
> organism to be his Self. He does not care to know that these are only
> instruments for the life of the Atman—his real Self on the material
> plane. So he indulges in gross physical pleasures. The desire for them
> becomes so strong that he becomes their victim. He does not enjoy
> them; they enjoy him.[9]

How many times have you felt like a victim of your own drives for sense pleasure, knowing you shouldn't indulge in something, yet being compelled to do
it anyway?

One of the components of subtle body is the unconscious. Yoga views the
unconscious similarly to depth psychologists such as Freud and Jung, as the repository of past experiences and the driving force behind much of an individual's

current actions and thoughts. The subtle body is held to exist independently of the physical body and doesn't undergo death as does the physical body. It contains the karmic impressions, desires, and tendencies developed over the course of countless lifetimes, not just one lifetime as thought by Western psychology.

These impressions, called *samskaras,* which I mentioned earlier, are stored in the subtle body and determine much of what we do, seek, and experience in this life. Kshemaraja writes, "The various desires of such a person are awakened by the force of his subtle body, and he wanders from life to life by acquiring suitable bodies in which these desires can be suitably satisfied."[10] The mind creates the physical body for the purposes of experiencing the results of past actions (karma) and for the fulfillment of current desires on the material plane. Those notions concerning the nature of the mind and its existence from one life to the next are in direct contradiction to these basic assumptions of traditional Western psychology: (1) the physical body is the only body that we have, (2) death is the inevitable end of human existence, and (3) physical death is the final termination of human consciousness.[11]

The yogic conceptualization of the unconscious differs from Freud's view in terms of how the contents of the unconscious arrive there. Freud held that repression is the process by which most of the content of the unconscious is created, whereas yoga psychology asserts that practically every thought, desire, act, or experience leaves its trace regardless of whether or not it's repressed. These traces, the samskaras, built up over time, serve as templates or potentialities for the creation of future thoughts, desires, actions, and bodies.

Yoga psychology takes a very practical approach toward remedying the problems of the mind. Given that past impressions have been deposited over innumerable lives, it is impossible to search for all the antecedent causes determining our present psychological make-up. There's no point to endlessly searching our past and analyzing traumas. Such a search would be fruitless in terms of stilling the mind and preventing the continued influence of those impressions. Since the basic problem is root ignorance of who we truly are and the subsequent modifications of the mind—the thoughts, emotions, and the deluded ideas of who we are—then the solution is the stilling of the modifications of the mind and the eradication of the root ignorance.

All yoga practices aim at stilling the mind and eradicating the root ignorance. Patanjali, writes in the Yoga Sutras, "When the mind is still then man abides in his true nature."[12] To enable one to abide in one's true nature, yoga examines and classifies the contents of the mind and prescribes remedies, the yogic practices, for reducing and eliminating the thought waves, or modifications of the mind.

All modifications of the mind, called *vrittis,* can be classified as one or a combination of five types and categorized as either painful or non-painful. The five types are: right knowledge, wrong knowledge, fantasy, deep sleep, and memory. *Painful* and *non-painful* have special meanings in the yoga context. Painful vrittis refer to thought waves that manifest or sustain the delusion that we are not the Self. Thus, sense pleasures, even your favorite chocolate cake or whatever else you take delight in, are considered painful because they reinforce ideas such as "I am the body, the source of my joy is external, my identity is limited in some way, love comes from this or that." Such vrittis produce desires, causing us to search for some objects while avoiding others, which keep us bound to the cycle of birth and death. Non-painful vrittis are of either a neutral type, such as simply perceiving the sky as you're walking, or of the type that lead toward liberation and identification with our true Self, for example thoughts such as, "I am not limited to the body, I am not limited to the mind, I am the Self."

Notice that the two broad categories are "painful" and "non-painful," not "painful" and "pleasurable" or "joyful." It's a very important point. It reflects the yogic insight that modifications of the mind, no matter what type, do not produce true pleasure, joy, or love. The qualities of joy and love, called *ananda,* are infinite dimensions of the Self. Yoga asserts that as we split ourselves off from our innate ananda, our ecstasy, our Self, we then project it onto objects and people and seek it externally. We build up the belief that joy will really come from eating rich, creamy, chocolate-chocolate-chip ice cream! Our minds become agitated with the desire for it. When we finally walk to the store, come home, and dig into it, there's a moment when the desire ceases, the mind is still, and we're in the bliss of chocolate, chocolate chip! "No!" says the yogi! We're in the bliss of our own Self (ananda), which we've experienced a reflection of the moment when our mind was still—free of thoughts and desires. The yogic perspective holds that joy and love always arise from within. If joy were really in the chocolate ice cream, then every time we ate it, and no matter how much we ate, we would experience that joy, just as we experience the coldness and chocolateness that really are qualities of the ice cream. We delude ourselves into believing that pleasure, love, and joy are qualities of the world rather than seeing them as arising from the source within and turning our attention toward the Self, immersing ourselves in our innate center of love, allowing it to flow outward as naturally as a rose shares its beauty and fragrance with all passersby.

THE MIND'S DELUDED NATURE

The process by which we become deluded is essentially a conditioning process very similar to the conditioning processes described in modern cognitive-behavioral psychology. The sequence in the conditioning process is (1) avidya, the primal ignorance manifested as the identification with the limited self instead of the true Self creates the mental agitation of desire, obscures our real nature and the experience of all-encompassing wholeness and bliss inherent to it; (2) the desires are focused on a particular object; (3) possession of the object temporarily eliminates the agitation caused by the desires, thus allowing the mind to be relatively still; (4) in that stillness, the joy or feeling of completeness that is our true nature arises within us. This feeling is temporally paired with the object, and we erroneously come to believe that the object gave rise to the joy or pleasure.

We're particularly susceptible to conditioning because we are primarily identified with our subtle and physical bodies. Our attention is focused on sensory and mental-emotional events and their co-occurrences. The causal body and the Self are beyond the effects of conditioning. In their respective states of deep sleep and turiya, conditioning cannot occur. In deep sleep we're not aware of any physical or mental events, and in turiya we're beyond them. Yoga practices can be viewed as deconditioning practices aimed at breaking the conditioning patterns established through lifetimes of identification with our minds and bodies. Stephen Wilson, PhD, described the processes by which one becomes a yogi as resocialization and deconditioning processes.[13] Thus, research on advanced yogis and Zen masters has shown that in some states, they don't habituate to stimuli or they don't react at all, both of which interfere with the conditioning process. Because of their effectiveness in deconditioning, yoga practices, primarily meditation, are used clinically in application to stress reactivity, psychosomatic illnesses, and anxiety disorders. However, it must be remembered that the level of deconditioning that they were originally aimed at is deeper and broader than those therapeutic applications imply. Daniel Goleman, PhD, writes:

Asian psychologies have largely ignored psychologically loaded contents of awareness, including psychodynamics, while seeking to alter the context in which they—and all other information—are registered in awareness. Conventional psychotherapies assume as givens the mechanisms underlying perceptual, cognitive, and affective processes, while seeking to alter them at the level of socially conditioned patterns. Asian systems disregard these same socially conditioned patterns, while aiming at the control and self-regulation of the underlying mechanisms themselves. Therapies break the hold of past conditioning on present behavior; meditation aims to alter the process of conditioning per se so that it will no longer be a prime determinant of future facts. In the Asian approach behavioral and personality change is secondary, an epiphenomenon of changes, through the voluntary self-regulation of mental states, in the basic processes which define our reality.[14]

All modifications of the mind are to be overcome by intense practice and detachment born of discrimination. In yoga, discrimination is the ability to differentiate between the Self and the mind, between one's true nature and one's assumed, limited nature, between the Infinite and the finite. With that ability, one can detach from the desires and conditioned identity of the mind and body. The intense practice refers to the eight types of yogic disciplines—yamas, niyamas, asana, pranayama, pratyahara, dharana, dhyana, and samadhi—referred to as the eight limbs of yoga (we'll look at these in more detail in chapter 10). They are aimed at reducing and eventually eliminating all the current modifications of the mind, as well as all the samskaras from the past. These practices and the yogic process they engender purify the subtle body of all the impressions of past lifetimes and eventually destroy avidya, the root ignorance of one's essential nature.

The practices don't improve the Self or change the Self. The Self isn't bound and the Self can't be liberated. The mind, however, is bound. Vedanta likens the mind to a dirty mirror, and its power to reflect reality is obscured and distorted. Yogic practices remove the dirt, the vrittis, and then the purified mind reflects the luminous Consciousness of the Self. Patanjali warns aspirants that they need to be prepared to practice yoga for lifetimes in order to be established in the highest samadhi that pervades the waking, dream, and deep sleep states.

Yoga psychology shows that the mind takes the form of whatever it dwells on, like water taking the shape of any container into which it is poured. Normally our mind is focused on the subtle and physical bodies, taking their forms and identifying with them. Thus, consciousness is ordinarily limited to the body and mind and the roles and functions they perform. In the process of meditation, the mind is withdrawn from the physical body and directed toward the pure boundless Consciousness of the Self. The mind dwelling on the formless Self dissolves its limited nature and becomes one with Consciousness. All vrittis cease, and one abides in one's true nature, to paraphrase Patanjali. Repeated immersion in samadhi purifies one of all samskaras, all the past impressions of limitations, and shifts one's identity from the mind-body complex to pure Consciousness. When we're identified with our minds, we think of our limited self as the subject, the knower, the perceiver of objects. During the course of yoga, it becomes clear that the body, the mind, and all its contents, as well as the states of waking, dreaming, and deep sleep, are objects of perception for a conscious knower. That conscious knower, which is never an object of knowledge, is the Self.[15] It is always the Seer, never seen. Ultimately one's identity remains established in one's Self even in the midst of all the thoughts and actions of the conventional self, the ego mind.

When I did my research project for my doctoral degree at Temple University in 1984–86, I chose to study the effects of long-term practice of an awakened Kundalini-based yoga. The study looked at three groups of people, each representing a different style of practice, with all the individuals having practiced for more than ten years. One group was comprised of swamis—renunciate monks living in an ashram—and another group was made up of people living in an ashram but not monks. The third group was comprised of householders—people practicing in the midst of family life and work demands.

What I found was that awakened Kundalini had an impact on virtually every aspect of people's lives. The groups were nearly identical in how they experienced the changes. There turned out to be seven broad categories of change: physical, emotional, mental, relational, conceptual, attitudinal, and values and priorities. There were 169 types of changes across those categories that impacted everything from how one's body is perceived, to self-concept, attitudes towards oneself, others and the world, and changes in understanding what the meaning and purpose of having a human birth are. You can see by the comprehensiveness of the categories of change that everything about these practitioner's lives was transformed as a result of shaktipat and Kundalini awakening.[16]

Awakened Kundalini purifies the physical and subtle bodies of all blocks, the samskaras, and hidden mental tendencies and eliminates the primal ignorance (avidya), which causes bondage. Because it works at the most fundamental level, it impacts all levels of mind-body functioning, thus it impacts our whole lives. Shakti becomes the motive power behind all the practices of yoga—the yamas, niyamas, asana, pranayama, and so forth—and takes the aspirant to the goal of liberation. The purification work of Kundalini Shakti goes beyond anything the ego mind is capable of and results in the unity state of consciousness, where all distinctions between the Infinite and finite, God and Self, the material and nonmaterial world all dissolve and paradoxically remain, but only on the level at which such differences have their ephemeral existence.

It is to the ultimate state that the eternal quest points. Kundalini awakening and unfolding are the means for success on this highest quest. The soul's yearning for freedom, joy, love, and delight is an expression of our true Self calling us home. Living in a state of wisdom and grace allows the Divine to infuse all of our activities with love and compassion. It's not an attainment that is meant only for renunciates, monks, and monastery or ashram dwellers, but for everyone. In India there is a rich tradition of householder saints, men and women of the highest attainment, who lived family lives and worked as potters, shoemakers, weavers, farmers, and teachers. We need such models of an integrated life of the full Consciousness.

Kundalini awakening is often accompanied by more and more energy pouring into the mind and body. The practices and the disciplines of yoga, meditation, seva, and fulfilling the dharma—the responsibilities of one's life—help to form and strengthen the inner container for what can be to the ego mind a tumultuous, powerful coursing energy. Stabilizing the mind and body through these practices is an essential part of being empowered to traverse one's path. It gives the ego mind what it needs to engage in as right effort, as a way of coming into harmony with, and surrendering to the unfolding of your boundless nature. You have to be able to cultivate the practices that strengthen the mind and body and their ability to be present with increasing energy.

When I get calls and emails from people, whether they are reaching out to me from New Zealand, Germany, Great Britain, Canada, Australia, or other places around the world, it's usually something like this: "There's too much energy, what do I do? I've had a Kundalini awakening, and there's too much energy going on. It's disrupting my life. I need help." That's the natural cry of the ego mind when suddenly it's confronted with this boundless energy, and it does need help. Even yogis find themselves unprepared for what can happen with Kundalini awakening. Your essential nature is boundless, its energy is boundless, its power is boundless, and its love is boundless; its intuition, its wisdom, these are all boundless. As the ego mind begins to catch the first waves of that boundlessness (no boundaries), it's not unusual for it to feel challenged or swept off balance. The ego mind needs healthy boundaries to optimally function and serve as it is designed to serve.

There are practices that help the ego mind and strengthen it in positive ways, ways that don't strengthen its clinging, don't strengthen its fear, don't strengthen its anger and its reactivity, but strengthen its steadiness, strengthen its ability to be present as a servant. That's what Kundalini sadhana, the practices and process of Kundalini awakening and unfolding, does for the ego mind. When the mind is feeling tumultuous, whether it's in our emotional life or in the energy of the body or the periods of chaos in everyday living, we can learn to use the tools Kundalini Shakti gives us to bring our attention and our mind back to a calmer and steadier place. One of these practices is a *dharana*, a type of focused meditation practice in which you focus on entering the steady awareness of a mountain. Accessing this steady state is invaluable for moving through life with greater ease and strength.

Doing this type of practice and other yogic and meditative practices with discipline and regularity is necessary for integrating experiences, staying on track with Kundalini's dance, and navigating the mysterious and at times treacherous phases when the mind is in the cloud of unknowing.

MOUNTAIN DHARANA

Doing this meditation practice routinely will develop your capacity for steady awareness and unshakeable rootedness.

Begin by coming into your best meditation posture, a posture that is comfortable and at ease, supporting full and effortless breathing. Simply follow the breath, allowing your attention to rest on the breath. Your awareness will begin to detach and step back as you're just watching the movement of the breath, the movement of the mind, allowing the body to settle. Your attention is resting inside. As your breath settles, the mind begins to settle. Allow it to simply rest on the waves of the breath for a while.

Shift your attention to the sense of the heaviness of your body resting at ease. Every breath is an invitation to the body and the mind to let go and let go. Your awareness is just watching, detached and at ease, spacious and free.

Letting go and letting go clears the space for now imagining a majestic mountain. It may be a mountain that you've seen or are familiar with, a mountain that you've only seen a picture of, or a mountain that just occurs in your imagination at this time. It is a magnificent mountain, strong and steady. And as you're watching that mountain, it's as if you can feel the power, the steadiness of that mountain, the rootedness of that mountain that extends down into the earth, to its unshakable core. At the same time, the mountain rises up into the heights, the mountain stands steady, majestic in its grandeur.

Imagine that you're sitting on that mountain, comfortably sitting on the side of the mountain, feeling that steadiness beneath you. Allow your awareness to sink down into that mountain, into that steadiness feeling, the unshakeable quality of that mountain. Sense the mountain awareness, unmoved, unmoving. Winds may blow, storms may come and go, and yet that mountain stands steady in its grandeur, its majesty untouched, unshakeable. And you inhale deeply that steadiness, that majesty and grandeur of your mountain nature.

Drawing it into every cell of your body, you can feel that deep rootedness, a rootedness that also supports life, just as a great mountain may have villages and the lives of countless creatures that depend on it. But still, its unshakeable, steady quality is forever present. Allow that steadiness, the awareness and the feeling of that to sink into the body, all the way down into your bones, so every cell in your body feels supported and strengthened with that unshakeable steadiness. You're rooted, rooted in that mountain nature, your majestic, grand nature as a magnificent being, as who you truly are.

Inhale that fully and deeply, and feel the radiance of that permeate your body, giving it strength and steadiness, unshakeable confidence. You can face anything; you remain rooted in the truth of who you are, your sublime Self. You're rooted in your true nature. You can come back to that awareness of unshakeable rootedness over and over again, rest there for as long as you like. Take refuge in that awareness, an awareness that reflects the truth of your steady powerful presence, unshakeable and true.

8

Finding and Following the Truth through Viveka, Discrimination

The Shiva Sutras say simply that a seeker is one who makes an effort. Everyone receives grace. The seeker makes the right effort as well. Right effort includes the moment-by-moment application of discrimination, the ability to differentiate between what is true and what isn't. The seeker must be vigilant about applying their discrimination—this is part of being awake, aware, and clear. We use our discrimination in sadhana to examine the mind and the ego, and we look closely into where thoughts, feelings, sensations, attitudes, and impulses arise from and where they will take us. Right effort means we fully engage in sadhana. We commit to practicing and studying the philosophy and psychology of meditative and mystical traditions. In sadhana one calls on the power of the practices, such as meditation, mantra, pranayama, contemplation, or other practices, and integrates them into everyday life. On the path to radical freedom, there is no time off from sadhana. Sadhana doesn't stop when the meditation timer goes off or when we stop repeating a mantra or come off our yoga mat. It includes all the joys, love, passion, delight, challenges, and pains of life.

Not long after meeting Muktananda, I was off on an adventure with a friend who took me spelunking. I had no idea I was about to encounter the power of mantra practice on this outing. I had never been in any deep caves before and now I was part of a small team led by a geology professor. We were going into a barely explored cave that was at the bottom of a hundred-foot sinkhole in a forest in upstate New York.

It was nighttime when we arrived, so we were repelling straight down into the abyss in the dark! It didn't matter that it was nighttime, the professor said, because inside the cave it would be absolutely pitch black even at noon on a sunny day. We had headlamps, helmets, ropes, water, all the gear for exploring the cave. We were going to be in for a few hours and then come out. A small stream ran along the bottom of many of the cave's passage ways. These winding tunnels were so small in places that I often had to crawl or walk hunched over. Bats clung to the ceilings in the first part of the cave, but as we went deeper and deeper we left them behind. It was pouring rain outside when we were repelling down so there was more water than the professor expected.

I had done rock climbing, hiking, and mountain climbing in the past, but doing these things in the pitch dark was amazing. When we all shut our little headlamps off, it truly was so dark you couldn't see your fingers touching your nose. The weird echoes off the rocks were disorienting in the black cavern and nearly made me dizzy. The cave floor was pitched downward, forcing us to descend deeper into the earth as we continued onward. Getting out would be all uphill and then a hundred-foot straight-up ascent to get out of the sinkhole. It was already after midnight at this point.

We came to a small tunnel leading off the main route and my friend suggested to the professor that we explore it. The professor told my friend and I and a couple of other people to go ahead and do that and then meet them back in the larger tunnel in an hour. My friend suggested I lead the way into the tunnel. The tunnel got narrower and narrower, eventually reaching a point where I had to slither on my belly like a snake. My friend said he thought the tunnel opened up again further down so I kept going. We were slithering along in the mud and gravel as a little streamlet ran along the bottom of the tunnel. It was cold and wet and so narrow that I couldn't even raise my head enough to look further down the tunnel. All I could do was stare at the mud just inches from my face. Suddenly it dipped down and back up, like the bends in a piece of drainpipe that form a trap, and I managed to somehow get through it, inch by inch, summoning all my yogic flexibility! But then a few feet further down, the tunnel narrowed so much I couldn't go another inch. The rough rock walls pressed in all around me.

To my horror, I discovered that no one else had made it through the bend in this stone tunnel that I was now stuck in alone. I couldn't hear them, they couldn't hear me, and then my light went out. My arms were pinned down along my sides, and there wasn't enough room to even inch them over my head. I was lying cold and wet in a stone straightjacket two hundred feet below the surface. Then I began wondering what would happen if rain filled the tunnel I was now clogging. That's when my body and mind really began to panic. My poor body began to shake with fear.

Mantra saved my life. As I brought my mind back to the mantra Om Namah Shivaya, breath after breath, silently repeating it while lying face down in the rocks and water, it completely absorbed my attention. It was almost like I was in a meditation cave. Gradually my breath began to slow and deepen. My mind began to quiet and clear. My body relaxed and warmed. I was ready to discover what I could do to extricate myself from that very deep hole. I had to shimmy backwards, uphill, feet first, on the rocks, in the mud and water, barely making a quarter of an inch at a time. There was no other choice.

My poor body was exhausted, it was about 2:00 a.m., and I had no idea how long it would take to get out. Navigating the down- and up-bends in the tunnel, backwards, feet first, pinned to the floor without even enough room to turn onto my back, took all my strength. After discovering that my light went out because I hit the switch when my helmet hit the cave ceiling (which was only a foot from the cave floor!), I found I could turn it on as well. I kept it off because I didn't know how long the battery would last or how long I would be trapped. I took refuge in the mantra countless times as I worked my way out of that darkest of deep black holes. Om Namah Shivaya never failed me, never.

Though it felt like an eternity, it was probably a couple more hours before I made it back to the main tunnel of the cave, found the others, and we worked our way out of there. It turned out none of them were very experienced cavers, not even the professor. They had convinced themselves that I was just off exploring on my own and were shocked to hear otherwise. We got back to the surface at dawn.

I retreated to my tent totally exhausted. There was so much for me to contemplate, to examine what happened and what it meant in my sadhana. There were plenty of obvious lessons about caving, the dangers involved and the need for a real expert guide, but I was much more focused on sadhana. The experience dramatically showed the power of mantra to get me through even life-threatening circumstances. Absorbing my mind in the mantra kept it free of fear. The power of the mantra enveloped me and allowed the mind and body to function at their best to get me free from the stone-cold grip of the tunnel that otherwise might have become my tomb. The practices support us every step of the way in Kundalini sadhana. Our sadhana, empowered by Kundalini's grace, enables us to discriminate between the noise of the mind and steady wisdom of the Self calling us home, regardless of how lost in the darkness we may become.

In time, with dedicated self-discipline, the practices arise on their own, drawing you back to the truth of who you are; the breath calms and deepens on its own; the mantra fills you day and night; the throb of pure Consciousness that is the essence of mantra remains ever-present. Becoming deeply immersed in the practices and the wisdom of discernment is made easier with the right supports: the Three Jewels, self-effort, a commitment to awakening, and self-discipline.

THE THREE JEWELS

On the path of Kundalini everyone needs support. It is not a do-it-yourself project; in fact, no serious spiritual path is. Twenty-five hundred years ago Buddha spoke about the Three Jewels, also known as the three refuges, as the necessary supports that seekers need. Just as a step stool must have three legs in order for one to stand on it, these three elements provide the steady support needed to traverse the path. One is a wise and accomplished teacher; another is the support of the practices, writings and the disciplines of the path; and the third is the support of like-minded seekers, the *sangha,* a community of people dedicated to the practices and teachings. These three supports are the optimal way to sustain ourselves on our path of increasing wakefulness. Buddha's teachings on the Three Jewels give a broad understanding of what is necessary to complete the heroic journey of sadhana.

Buddha also said if those supports aren't available, it doesn't mean you abandon practice; you go on even in the face of the additional challenges. The prison inmates I had the good fortune to practice with showed what extraordinary fruit comes to those who continue with their sadhana even when all the supports aren't ideally present. There's an inspiring book about practicing without all of the supports, *Dharma In Hell,* by Fleet Maull, which I highly recommend.

He speaks of being an inmate while practicing and teaching Buddhism in prisons for many years.

On the path of Kundalini, a practitioner needs the support of highly qualified and experienced teachers, fellow practitioners, practices, and sources of knowledge and wisdom that help the mind act in harmony with the transformative power of Kundalini.

FOCUSED USE OF SELF-EFFORT

Along with the Three Jewels, fully engaged sadhana also requires dedicated self-effort. You can have the great good fortune to have a wise and selfless teacher, the support of teachings and practices available, and a wonderful community of committed practitioners, but without self-effort, transformation may slow to a halt. Right effort engages the mind in a positive way. Even while Kundalini's grace is transforming your entire life, the mind is always asking, what do I do? How do I deal with Kundalini? The ego mind is an organ for doing things in the world. We need to find the off-switch for the ego mind in order to discover what happens when it finally ceases its doing and trying. It's also necessary to bring the ego mind's efforts into harmony with what Kundalini is unfolding. It needs to learn what comprises right effort and skillful action. Three critical areas for applying self-effort are sadhana practices, sustaining optimal physical and mental health, and finding and working with a qualified teacher.

SADHANA PRACTICES

Sadhana practices include all the classic yoga and meditation practices that, for example, are included in Patanjali's Ashtanga yoga (see chapter 10) or Buddha's Noble Eightfold Path or the various means and methods for knowing the highest from other comprehensive spiritual traditions. Sadhana as a whole encompasses all of the three areas of self-effort. Classic sadhana practices focus on typical spiritual or yogic practices. Awakened Kundalini spontaneously adds to these traditional practices and refines them by emphasizing some at one time and others at another time. There may be periods when Shakti pulls you into meditation for hours a day, and at other times there's much less meditation and more hatha yoga, seva, chanting, or studying texts for contemplation. In Kundalini sadhana, discerning the directions Shakti is giving you is of paramount importance. In the face of uncertainty or doubt, not knowing what

Shakti is asking of you, you rely on the dharma of your spiritual path and the guidance of your teacher.

There are several critically important areas where we need to be especially conscious and awake as we do our sadhana practices and develop our discrimination. They are

1. discerning the way of Truth through discrimination,
2. self-discipline,
3. optimizing physical and mental health,
4. studying with a qualified teacher, and
5. commitment to awakening and remaining awake.

DISCERNING THE WAY OF TRUTH THROUGH DISCRIMINATION

In this process of Kundalini unfolding, we cultivate attitudes and ways of relating to the mind, the body, others, and the world, all of which are informed by Kundalini's view. Kundalini sees the truth at all times and in all places. Developing discrimination is of primary importance in sadhana because it removes the distorted lens of ignorance, which prevents us from seeing clearly. This distortion is what leads to all forms of suffering. Later we'll examine additional qualities and attitudes that are cultivated in elements of the eight limbs of Classical yoga and the Buddha's Noble Eightfold Path.

Viveka: Discrimination

Kundalini sadhana, as well as all yoga sadhanas, demands the careful cultivation of discrimination, or *viveka*, the ability to discern the difference between what's true and what isn't, between Self and self, between the Infinite and the finite. Viveka cuts the root of avidya, the primal ignorance of your true nature that gives rise to all suffering and countless cycles of death and rebirth. On the highest level, discrimination empowers you to see the Divine everywhere, as everything, and as your own true nature—One without a second. With that vision, you embrace all as your dearest Self, love flows with abandon, and patience and compassion give unction to all. Ultimate discrimination comes naturally, effortlessly, from the sublime state of the Self.

The *paramahamsa*, the great swan, is an ancient symbol of discrimination in the Vedic tradition. It is said that the paramahamsa has such powers of discrimination that when milk is mixed with water, the paramahamsa can drink the milk alone, leaving behind the water. The milk symbolizes the pure knowledge of the Divine, mixed with every moment, but obscured to those without the discrimination to see it and draw from it. Every moment is an opportunity to practice discrimination, to differentiate what is true from what is untrue—including and most importantly, the truth of who you are and what the nature of all beings and all creation is.

As Kundalini gives one the direct experience of that truth, it sharpens one's discrimination and allows one to see what is *sat,* Sanskrit for what is true, at all times in all places, and what is *asat,* false or not true. It may be true some of the time or in some places, but not all the time in all places. Viveka is the ability to differentiate between the two, even as thoroughly mixed as they are in each moment, including this moment. What is eternal, what is ephemeral, right now? Examine your immediate experience.

It is also viveka that allows you to differentiate between the promptings of ego and the wisdom arising from the Self, Pure Consciousness, Shakti. The Self has classically been described as having the qualities of *Satchitananda. Sat* means it is true in all times and places, eternally true. *Chit*, all-encompassing Consciousness, is another of its irreducible qualities, as is *ananda*—ecstasy, uncaused, ever-present bliss suffused with all-embracing Love. Kundalini sadhana demands that one has the discrimination to know how Shakti is uniquely guiding one's practices toward direct knowledge of Satchitananda, your true Self. Avidya, the root ignorance, confuses the self with the Self. Thus, we identify with the ephemeral, continuously constructed false self, the ego mind, and dis-identify with the Self that is sat, eternally true.

Kundalini sadhana turns every moment, every action of the mind or body into a practice. Kundalini illumines whether you are doing practices that further reveal and reflect your Divine Self or obscure and cloak it, right here, right now. We can bring greater discrimination into any moment by asking ourselves: What am I identified with? What have I become in this moment? The body, feelings, sensations, roles we play—we become these so effortlessly, so habitually, and compulsively that we lose consciousness of our Self. Every time we think, "I am happy" or "I am annoyed" or "I am challenged," whatever the "I am ____" is, we've bound our consciousness to that particular thing. Discrimination allows us to see it and let it go, even if the feeling remains. It's the mind's feeling or the body's feeling; it doesn't bind and limit you. You are pure, Infinite Consciousness. You can see the mind and its content, and discern where it came from and how limited it is. The mind is powerless to affect your true nature. Discrimination on an absolute level makes this clear.

On the everyday level of practice, the mind's discrimination has to become more and more refined in order to follow Kundalini without getting lost in delusion. In Kundalini sadhana, you have to be able to differentiate between what is arising from the mind caught in ignorance and what is arising from the wisdom of Kundalini. Discrimination gives us the clarity to know when an impulse is a movement of Shakti to be followed and when it is a samskara, an old impression or pattern that Shakti is bringing up to be released. Cultivating discrimination sharpens the mind and makes it more facile. These are critical strengths to have for navigating the subtle and fluid course of Kundalini. There are countless ways you will use your discrimination.

One fellow who contacted me for help asked about why he was feeling so driven to eat meat. He had become a vegetarian years earlier when he initially experienced Kundalini awakening and felt it had supported him being lighter, healthier, and clearer in his meditations. But now he was craving meat, thinking of ordering meat when he went to restaurants, even dreaming of eating meat. He wasn't suffering any ill health or negative side effects from his vegetarian diet. In fact, he was very good about eating a well balanced diet with all the protein and nutrition that he needed. It sounded to me as if the samskaras of craving and needing meat were being flushed out, and it would be best to detach from them, let them go and become free from them. Clearly he was identifying with the desires. "They're *my* desires; I *feel* this way; I *feel* compelled to eat meat," was what he said. He became so thoroughly identified with the desires that they finally drove him to eat meat. Buddha said, "as you think, so you become."

He discovered that eating meat made him feel heavy, and it ruined his digestion. He felt lethargic and dull in meditation. He said it was like the wonderfully energizing fire of yoga that he had been feeling was nearly extinguished. He stopped eating meat and in time the energy returned. The cravings reappeared and lasted for months, but with the wisdom he gained from the experience, he remained detached. They finally faded away. I've also seen similar circumstances where the person was being pushed by Kundalini to eat meat, or fish, or rich foods, and it improved their health, vitality, and meditation. With Kundalini, you have to discern what is needed in the present for you and know that could change completely at another time in your sadhana. Discerning the difference between strong desires and guidance from Kundalini takes patience and surrender along with the Three Jewels.

The *Viveka-Chudamani* (Crest Jewel of Discrimination) by Adi Shankara, the same author of the *Saundaryalahari* quoted earlier, is one of the essential texts for understanding discrimination and how to apply it in sadhana. In addition, studying the principle texts of Kashmir Shaivism will deepen one's appreciation of Kundalini and develop one's discrimination, particularly for discerning the ways of Kundalini Shakti.

Discrimination has to be applied in looking at what comes up within ourselves and when evaluating the teachings and teachers that are being presented to us. We use our discrimination to tell if something is true and whether the impulse, intuition, insight, or vision is coming from the Self/Shakti or the ego mind. It's said in the yogic tradition that to know something is true, it must be validated by one's teacher, the sacred texts and teachings of one's tradition, and by one's own experience. It is the responsibility, or the dharma, of a seeker or practitioner of any tradition to develop their discrimination through study, contemplation, practice, and through interactions with their teachers and fellow practitioners.

What often challenges people's discrimination the most is their own pain. Whether it is pain that is part of one's life history or pain that one is going through as part of one's spiritual transformation, seeking an end to pain makes people vulnerable. It does this in ordinary relationships and relationships with teachers, gurus, lamas, priests, and others who seem to offer a way out of the pain. Some of these teachers may not deserve the level of trust and obedience the seeker in pain gives them. Empower yourself with discrimination. A true teacher empowers people and relieves suffering. They support people awakening and bringing their wakefulness into their lives with greater joy, love, compassion, patience, service, energy, and creativity.

Intense sexual energy also overwhelms people's discrimination and self-control. This is particularly evident as Kundalini moves through the lower chakras and may vastly intensify a seeker's sexual drives for some time. The container built by dedication to the practices and dharma must be strong enough to hold the energy. This energy can challenge marriages, relationships, and the teacher-student relationship. The great sage Patanjali said the teacher needs to be one who has risen above attachment and passion; they need to be free in order to guide the student through the maze of karmas and energies to a state of freedom. Even if the teacher loses their discrimination, hold onto yours.

Kundalini and tantra are sometimes used to camouflage both teachers' and seekers' raw sexual energy and desire with which they are so attached and identified. They become additional excuses for acting out and binding one to the karmas born of attachment to and identification with the body. A teacher abusing students in this way brings harm to themselves and their students, even if the student doesn't feel abused. The pseudo-practice of tantric sex is neither a shortcut to freedom from suffering nor a necessary part of sadhana. For most, it is a trap that can take lifetimes to escape. You are empowered to use your discrimination to avoid this trap.

THE WISE KNOW
The wise know these three to be separate:
   wants, needs and Love.
By reducing their wants and needs,
   Love fills the spaciousness of their being.
They want only the end of suffering
   and the fullness of joy for all beings.
They need only that which enables them
   to fulfill their dharma.
They Love with abandon all of creation!
This is what it is to be wise.
This is what it is to be fully human.

Animals, even insects fight over territory, possessions and mates,
kill each other for food and are constantly wary of attack,
What makes you any different?
Distinguish yourself from these suffering life-forms.
You have a precious human birth,
   what are you doing with it?
Any creature can be angry, hurtful,
   fearful, and greedy.

> You, you can be compassionate, loving, kind,
>   patient and free.
> The world cries out for your humanity,
>   your wisdom, your grace.
>
> You are Tara.
> You are Kwan Yin.
> You are Mary.
> You are Jesus.
> You are Krishna.
> You are Buddha.
> You are Kali.
> *Tat Twam Asi!*
> Drop your masks, drop your delusions!
> Now!
>   KALIDAS[1]

SELF-DISCIPLINE: DISCRIMINATION'S PARTNER

Self-discipline aligns your actions with your vision. Both will be tested over and over again throughout sadhana. For example, is Shakti calling you to change the company you keep, or is it fear and avoidance? Are the physical symptoms you are experiencing due to Kundalini, or do you have a medical condition? Is Kundalini making you sexually active, or is it confronting you with samskaras, old patterns, to sit through with detached equanimity as it sets you free? Discrimination develops from the light of Consciousness illuminating the essential difference between being true to your highest nature or not. One way leads to greater freedom, one to continued bondage.

The ordinary mind actually needs to routinely practice checking in with your highest nature, your Buddha mind, your Self or Higher Power by literally asking in the moment what that overarching dimension of your being sees or advises at that time. In any given situation, we can take a step back internally, detaching our awareness from the automatic view of the ego and ask our Self, our Buddha mind, for greater wisdom, clearer vision, inspired action, or simply to open to the spaciousness of awareness and stillness, inviting our true nature to express itself. Some people develop an image of their wise Self, whether it's an archetypal image of a wise old woman or man, or some other inspirational image. The ordinary mind is used to just going by its old patterns of instincts, conditioning, and desires. It's on autopilot. In sadhana, we invite the Divine within to guide and direct the instrument it created, our mind-body, to serve in the best ways possible. In any situation we ask ourselves, how I can serve the highest to the best of my abilities in this moment? In this way we decondition the mind-body and come into alignment with the Divine in the moment.

By stepping back and using your discrimination to examine why you feel drawn to a teacher, a practice, a tradition, an experience, you discern what dynamics are affecting the mind-body, drawing it toward one thing or repelling it from another. You'll use your discrimination for discerning the best practices for you to be doing, for determining how Shakti responds to your diet, your lifestyle, relationships, every aspect of your life.

We have to use our discrimination to discern if what is happening is due to Kundalini's transformative processes or if what is happening is because of what we are doing. People have come to me complaining that Kundalini is ruining their health. When we examined the whole picture of what practices they were doing and what their lifestyle was like in order to discern what was affecting their Kundalini process, often a different picture would emerge. In one case, we discussed what they ate, what filled their mind, what kinds of meditative and contemplative practices they were doing, and what kinds of exercise and physical health practices they were following. As often happens, there were critical elements missing in their practices. It wasn't Kundalini that was challenging their health, but how they lived, acted, and reacted to life that was problematic.

Deep practice requires great self-discipline. Discipline refers to the order necessary to receive direction and instruction, in this case from Kundalini herself. A disciple is defined as one who willingly follows that order, that discipline. Become a disciple of your own inner power, of the Divine within. Become a disciple of your Kundalini. She will show you how your sadhana is affected by what you eat, what you feed the mind, what company you keep, how you promote the optimal health of your body, and how much you cultivate generosity and selflessness through service to others.

Discrimination empowers one to discern the difference between the pleasant and the good. There are practices, experiences, relationships, and other activities that are pleasurable, thus attractive to the ego mind, but they aren't

good for us from the standpoint of sadhana, of moving toward greater freedom from the conditioned mind. Our culture and the advertising world sell
a wide variety of ways to feel better, be sexier, have more confidence, be more
attractive by wearing certain clothes or driving a certain car, taking particular supplements, and on and on. In sadhana, seeking outside yourself for joy,
wholeness, and a fully expanded state of consciousness is the path to continued
bondage. The ego mind is so easily deluded by the promise of a shortcut to
feeling great, being free, or having power. This blind spot of the ego runs deep.
This is in part why it is helpful to check in with a trusted teacher and learn from
what other practitioners—past and present—have discovered. We now have a
vast collection of writings of great masters from many traditions that is more
accessible than anyone would have imagined just fifty years ago. The accessibility is a real boon as long as it's not a trap for the ego mind, which easily confuses
book knowledge for true wisdom and attainment.

Kundalini processes require especially high levels of self-control and integration accomplished in service of the Self. More energy is being released, and
Shakti, the enormous power of Consciousness, needs strong channels to run
through. The foundational practices are essential for doing that. Just as the
banks are to a river, so is self-discipline to Shakti flowing into the boundless
ocean of clear light awareness. If we don't have strong banks to guide the flow
of the great river of Shakti, then it's at risk of flowing all over the place. That's
when people feel like their mind is being flooded, things feel out of control,
and the ego mind feels frightened and struggles to integrate experiences or stay
grounded in everyday life.

It's really the discipline of the practices done regularly with genuine commitment and enthusiasm that strengthen the channels for that energy to flow
through and bring your consciousness back to its highest nature. That empha-
sis on discrimination and self-discipline, on doing the practices daily, is as
much a part of the unfolding of Kundalini as it might be in other disciplines
that one does. Daily foundational practices often include the cultivation of
compassion and lovingkindness, the use of mantra, mindfulness, selfless service to family and community, contemplation, meditation, aerobic exercise,
hatha yoga, and good nutrition.

The experience of radical freedom blossoms from being liberated from the
conditioned mind. What binds us is the ego mind, with its limited identification

and its conditioning to react and respond in automatic ways, both conscious and unconscious. These patterns don't reflect our greatest, highest, most sublime nature. If we're not free to be loving, kind, patient, and wise in every situation, then how much freedom do we have? If we're just acting out however we might have been programmed by past relationships, family, culture, or teachers, then we can only have a false sense of freedom. Awakening of Kundalini peels back all those layers that interfere with us being the fully free, compassionate, strong, wise, loving, kind, patient individual that we have the innate capacity to be in any situation. Discrimination allows you see when the ego mind is just spiritually posturing and when true wisdom and compassion are flowing through you. Discrimination clears your vision.

OPTIMAL PHYSICAL AND MENTAL HEALTH

The Shiva Sutras say that the body is the offering. We offer it in service to the Divine through sadhana. The body must be healthy and strong as a foundation for successful practice and as a foundation for a strong and healthy mind. The mind-body is our primary way of experiencing the world and engaging in sadhana. Cultivating physical and mental health and resilience are part of sadhana. In a sedentary society, we have to actually practice getting aerobic exercise, keeping the body strong and our prana moving. Eating a good, balanced diet free of toxins and processed foods is essential to sadhana. Fresh food is alive with prana that we take in when we eat it. Prana supports life and the unfolding of Kundalini's unique yoga.

Someone confronting health issues as part of their sadhana may have a physical therapist, surgeon, and doctor as supports for their sadhana. Another person may have a nutritionist and a psychologist on their team. Your sadhana supports are determined by what you need and how those needs change as Kundalini recreates your body, mind, and life.

Sadhana also includes watching what we feed the mind, what we pay attention to, steering clear of the constant bombardment of media and advertising in order to remain attentive to the Divine Presence, available to be moved by her quiet voice and subtle urgings. We feed the mind by the company we keep, both internally and externally. A seeker is very careful about the company he or she keeps. Studying the works of great masters, mystics, and poets feeds the mind and deepens one's wisdom. Keep the company of compassionate and wise masters through their writings. There may be times when old patterns arise in the mind that need to be worked through with the help of a psychologist or psychotherapist. That's simply another aspect of skillfully working to transform the mind.

Since Kundalini is the director of your sadhana, not the ordinary mind, being able to intuit, feel, or even hear her guidance and follow it demands a highly refined mind, a surrendered ego, and a body that can offer its best. Refining and strengthening the mind and body through the practices empowers one to follow her lead more and more gracefully, moment by moment.

Our physical and mental health are also directly linked to our relationships and work. Buddha spoke of right livelihood as that which causes no suffering to ourselves or others. Given the fragile nature of our global ecosystem we have to add being mindful of our impact on the environment. Conscious spirituality includes ecology as a part of right effort. Having work that is meaningful or is meaningful because of the attitude and awareness we bring to it supports greater congruence with the uplifting and transformative dynamics of Kundalini.

One woman who consulted me about her practices realized she needed to make many changes in her life to come into congruence with the direction that her true Self, through the power of Kundalini, was leading her. She had been a bartender for many years and, now in her forties, she needed to re-create her life. Her sadhana included getting career counseling, going back to school, and training in a new profession, in addition to the meditation, mantra, and selfless service practices she had been doing.

The same is true of relationships. Waking up impacts how clearly we see the relationships we're in and how they impact our sadhana. Sometimes we have to drop relationships and sometimes we have to drop attitudes and behaviors that prevent a relationship from being fully integrated into our sadhana. The use of discrimination is key for discerning what needs to happen.

STUDYING WITH A TEACHER

Finding a qualified teacher and receiving their guidance is another critical aspect of sadhana. It takes effort to find a good teacher; it takes more effort to regularly study with her or him and even more effort to overcome the hubris of the ego mind's many ways of telling itself it doesn't really need a guide or mentor, lama or guru. The ego mind loathes giving up its delusions, especially the one about its independence. In the absence of a selfless teacher who is skilled and knowledgeable about Kundalini, you have to exercise even more discrimination about what you study, where you receive instruction from, what you take in, and what tricks the ego mind is up to. Discrimination prevents one from giving over one's power because a teacher wears the right robes or is attractive in whatever way our ego mind finds attractive. Lifetimes can be wasted in wrong effort in this regard. This is part of why a wise and compassionate teacher is so highly valued in spiritual traditions.

COMMITMENT TO AWAKENING AND REMAINING AWAKE

Kundalini sadhana is all encompassing. Committing to awakening this inner power isn't the same as doing one practice—such as mindfulness training or yoga exercise for stress reduction, fitness, or well-being. Kundalini sadhana has one aim—the total radical freedom of complete enlightenment. Kundalini pursues that with one-pointed dedication and will strip the ego mind of all it clings to if that is the medicine required to free one from the bondage to limited selfhood and all the suffering it produces. Kundalini doesn't obey the ego mind; it doesn't follow a rational prescription of practices or processes that comforts the ordinary mind's need for a sense of control and predictability. For most people, Kundalini sadhana is a grace-filled process of expanding freedom and wakefulness. But for some it is a dramatically challenging process. And everyone on the path to radical freedom will at some point confront deep fears and attachments that are at the root of the ego mind.

The ego mind isn't in a position to determine the course of one's sadhana, though it can greatly influence how sadhana is experienced. When the ego mind aims to align itself with Kundalini through dedicated practice, sadhana flows more gracefully. Of course the ego can also choose to resist Kundalini by doing the opposite. In sadhana, it can often feel like the ego mind suffers from oppositional defiance disorder! You find your mind doing exactly what you know it shouldn't be doing! Yet fundamentally, Kundalini sadhana is the path of surrender to the will of the Divine, and we develop patience and compassion dealing with the ego and its resistance. Kundalini sadhana can be extremely challenging for the ego mind, but not for who you truly are. The source of transcendent wisdom and unshakeable support lies within you as you. Awakening to your true nature happens repeatedly; each time you forget, each time you fall asleep to the truth, the stage is set for re-awakening. When will you remain awake? Who can tell when the ripe fruit will fall? Your savritti phase has ended, the tide has changed, swim with the currents of Shakti!

Saraswati means "she who flows," and it is one of the most ancient terms for Kundalini. It's the fluid nature of this energy that clears the mind and body of these patterns that block us from knowing the truth of who we are and being able to live that truth moment by moment in every aspect of our lives. The heart is a boundless reservoir of compassion, patience, kindness, and love. Kundalini unlocks the full flow of these into your life. Because Kundalini is so fluid, you need great discrimination to discern her subtle and evolving ways of guiding your sadhana. We further develop that discrimination by clarifying the mind through meditation, chanting, mantra, contemplation, and selfless service.

VIVEKA EXERCISE

One of the classic ways of discriminating between the truth of who you are, the Self, and that with which you've identified yourself your entire life is to sit quietly, meditatively, and watch what arises in the mind, watch what arises in the inner sky of awareness.

Begin to notice that as something arises, be it a thought, a feeling, a sensation, a memory, or a fantasy, there's an impulse that arises with each of these that subtly asserts "that's me" or "that's mine." Now instead of allowing that assertion to go unchallenged, you will silently say to yourself, "not me, not mine" in response to anything and everything that arises in the spacious awareness. If you come to a place where nothing else arises, simply sit in that space of emptiness, of spacious awareness, for as long as you like. All the ephemeral things of the mind, with which the ego identifies, are empty of any permanence. Viveka, discrimination, allows you to see the difference between the forms and the emptiness they arise out of, and to see the difference between limited I-consciousness identified with "me" and "mine" and pure Consciousness free of all limitations.

9

Cultivating the Field for Awakening

Avidya and its product, ego identification, are at the root of suffering. Sadhana practices from all yogic and meditative traditions focus on dealing with the ego and its cause, avidya. One of the profound initial insights that emerges with awakening is that you are not your mind; you are not your ego. Many different meditative practices give you the experience of stepping back from the mind and seeing it for what it is. The distance and detachment that this insight brings gives you breathing room for working with the ego, seeing the ego mind and its ways of shaping reality and cultivating changes to the ego.

I vividly remember a woman in a meditation course I was teaching; she suddenly "got" this and blurted out, "You mean I don't have to follow my feelings!" Detaching from the mind grants you a measure of immediate freedom. It is part of what you can do to cultivate the field for awakening and for that awakening to mature and bear all its fruit.

Another valuable insight about the ego comes through the ancient wisdom of the Gnostic desert fathers. They said that if you see a person trying to climb to heaven on their own, pull them down. What the desert fathers were teaching is that if somebody is being solely driven by their ego, climbing as if self-effort alone would get them there, then they're destined for a fall. The sooner they come down, the sooner they will be able to correct their path and be less damaged from having climbed higher and fallen farther. The ego is easily impressed by its own efforts and believes them to be of paramount importance. Eventually Kundalini Shakti reveals how little the ego mind has accomplished with all its work compared with the total transformation wrought by grace. It is very humbling, crushingly so for the self-impressed ego. Fortunately, out of compassion She doesn't reveal this too early in sadhana or the ego might be daunted and give up.

As I mentioned in the previous chapter, we have to use our discrimination to see how the ego infiltrates all levels of practice and every perception of reality. Reining in the ego also involves opening our minds and hearts to the many kinds of support and help we need to traverse this path successfully. We rely on teachings, teachers, friends, books, music, and art, and that's in addition to all that we depend on simply to live: countless people, animals, insects, plants, earth, water, and the sun. There is no going it alone. We are completely interdependent. The ego's delusion of independence and rugged individualism make it blind and arrogant. It stumbles into one hole after another. Then as if it weren't trying to hide such a blunder, it acts as if it meant to fall in that hole. This is why we laugh at the "I meant to do that" line in comedy routines. We can see our own ego in it. In sadhana we have to retrain the ego mind and free it of such delusions. It will still make mistakes, but it doesn't have to scramble to cover them all the time. When the ego mind is grounded in the reality of its own limitations, there's a natural humility to it. Then it can gracefully serve the Divine within you and all of creation. It is particularly helpful to regularly contemplate our interdependence as an antidote to the ego's inflated state of delusion.

INTERDEPENDENCE CONTEMPLATION

In every moment, our complete interdependence with other people, other living creatures, plants, the elements, and even the sun and stars is evident. Pick up any thread of your existence and examine its connections. For example, look at your body. Every cell in your body had its origin elsewhere. Every atom in your body, in fact every atom of the whole earth, originated in a supernova billions of years ago. Every cell in your body is alive by the nourishment you've given it by the food you've eaten. Food made up of those same ancient atoms, food grown by others, harvested by others, transported by others, washed clean by others, perhaps even cooked by others. For that food to have grown, the right elements of water, air, sun, and soil had to come together under the careful eye of a farmer. Microbes had to make the nutrients available to the plant's roots. Bees had to pollinate the plant. Other insects, birds, and creatures helped the plant to grow. This is true of the plants that made the cloth for your clothes as well.

The interdependence grows exponentially when you consider all the beings that were involved with the production and delivery of the simplest of items in your life and the web of interdependencies that each of those beings is in. It is a complete illusion that we live separately, independently walking our path. All that we have exists in a web of interdependence, including all the wisdom and knowledge we will ever seek. With gratitude, we bow to all beings, all plants, and all the elements from the beginning of creation right up to this moment that make our life, our breath, and every facet of our existence possible. Each morning when you awake or before each meal, you can bring the great web of interdependence to mind with gratitude for all those who make your life possible.

EMPOWERED MEDITATION: KUNDALINI UNFOLDING

Directly knowing true freedom from the ego has two levels. On the absolute level, it is reuniting with the infinite expanse of Consciousness that is already present and has never been limited in any way by avidya and its creations, the ego mind and physical body. On a relative level, gaining freedom from the ego mind has to do with freedom from all the conditioned ways of acting and reacting, perceiving and receiving that make up our moment-by-moment existence.

Reducing the impact of the conditioned ego mind on the body and brain helps to free different parts of our neurophysiological system, like the amygdala, the part of the brain central to fear and anger, which are constantly triggered as part of our conditioned reactivity. This allows our entire body and nervous system to calm down, countering the stress response. This is why research on meditation and yoga shows reductions in blood pressure, stress hormones, cholesterol levels, headaches, and much more as these practices de-stress and decondition the reactivity of the mind and body. The neurophysiological research on meditators shows that the amygdala becomes less reactive and less easily provoked. These kinds of practices have a profound effect on our neuro-physiology, changing how our brain operates. Even as we free the mind of its conditioning, the mind is changing the brain and body, the physical organs of consciousness. H. H. the Dalai Lama's support of research in this area through the Mind and Life Institute and Dr. Richard Davidson's brilliant work and that of his colleagues at the University of Wisconsin–Madison are providing concrete scientific evidence on the power of meditative and contemplative practices to positively impact people's lives and even physically transform the brain.

In order to decondition the mind, we make use of foundational mindfulness practices by accessing the detached awareness that supports greater calm and equanimity. The ancient yogic tradition gives the ego mind something to do that's actually going to be helpful to reduce the conditioning instead of deepening it. We're used to having the ego mind engaged in the pursuit of all kinds of desires that it identifies with. Once one is on a path doing sadhana, the ego desires spiritual freedom, bliss, ecstasy, enlightenment, nirvana! What's it going to do, do, do? It is the organ of doing in the limited domain of ordinary reality. Thus, we give it practices that refine and develop its capacities to skillfully serve the living presence of the Divine, Kundalini's impulses, instead of its conditioned ones. In this way, you work with the basic tendency of the ego mind to "do" and bring it into alignment with cultivating qualities and practices that facilitate the awakening and unfolding of Kundalini.

Most of the practices from any meditative or yogic tradition are aimed at clarifying the mind, transforming it as an instrument of consciousness, and teaching it to abide in stillness—empowering the mind to be clear, quiet, and free of patterns of thought and reactivity. These practices also help to heal the body in ways that will allow body and mind to fully participate in the glory of your own nature, whether you think of that as your Buddha nature, Para Atman, Holy Spirit, Goddess within, or something else. It's really the transformation of the instruments of body and mind that the practices and the spontaneous events of Kundalini unfolding are all aimed at, in addition to cutting the root of avidya. Cutting the root is an act of grace. It is Shakti, the power of the Divine that created it, and it is solely by the grace of Shakti that bondage is severed.

One of the things that becomes clear in the course of sadhana is that we're either self-regulated or other-regulated. We're either in control of our mind, our attention, and our body, and in harmony with Shakti, or we're being led along by something external to ourselves or being driven by conditioning, by old patterns, habits, and impulses of the mind and body.

There's a growing body of scientific research looking at advanced meditators and yogis, as well as novices, that shows what happens to the mind and body as a result of practice. The research findings are helping to affirm the profound levels of deconditioning and added self-control and self-discipline that happen as a result of regular meditation and other contemplative/meditative practices. What happens when you immerse the mind in mantra? What happens when you repeatedly exercise the mind through mindfulness training? These practices have a profound impact on how your brain is operating, influencing your neurophysiology. These practices even change the thickness of the cortex in areas related to focus and attention. Yoga and meditative practices also diminish the deeply programmed fight-flight-freeze stress response in the body and mind. This is one of the most powerful conditioned responses that drive us and it undermines our physical and mental health. At an even deeper level is the brain pattern that's known as the habituation response, which is also overcome by meditation.

Habituation refers to the decreasing response to a stimulus that happens with repeated presentation of the stimulus. The classic example is the ticking clock that you first hear when you enter a room but within minutes you no longer do. It is still ticking, the stimulus is still present, but you've habituated to it and no longer respond to it by noticing the sound. The same thing happens to the sensation of the shoes on your feet, the watch on your wrist and many other things that are constantly stimulating our brain in some way but it shuts them out, saving our attention for more important stimuli. Habituation has long been thought of as a hardwired response, built into the neuro-circuitry of our brains.

Interestingly, back in the 1950s and '60s when research was beginning to be done on yogis, advanced meditators, and Zen masters, one of the findings that kept coming up was they were free to turn off the habituation response. Their practices freed them somehow from what was supposed to be hardwired and impossible to change. Researchers did a study in which they wired up a Zen master with sensors and they presented a click every fifteen seconds, watching to see when the brain would stop responding to it, because they could see a little blip in the EEG (electroencephalogram) every time the brain reacted to the sound. Untrained people will stop reacting within minutes due to habituation. Not the Zen meditators, they would just continue to be present, which makes sense since Zen meditation focuses on mindfulness, staying present in the moment and not tuning things out. Other meditation methods were examined as well, for instance a highly trained yogi was studied, and he was able to go into a state where he didn't react at all. At the same time his brain didn't show the kind of EEG that you would expect in sleep, for instance, when you're not responding to thunderstorms or sounds in your environment either.

The research showed that the brain has the capacity to either stay present with things that are consistently present, or step back from them, be aware but not reactive. This was mind-blowing for Western medicine at the time because the habituation response was part of what's called the autonomic nervous system (*autonomic* means automatic), and Western medicine thought the autonomic nervous system was not subject to volitional control. These things were all thought to be hardwired in, and yet here were yogis and advanced Zen masters doing things that set them free of even that deep level of conditioning, of what the mind-brain was evolutionarily set up to do to enhance survival.

If you wonder why the mind-brain evolved the habituation response, it has to do with attention. As humans were evolving and having to do everything necessary to survive, they needed all their resources available to pay attention to things that might be threatening in order to successfully run from it or fight it. We also evolved to have attention available to go after things that might be a food source or a potential mate. The attention mechanisms that our brain evolved were geared toward being available for those basic drives. Anything that is present in our environment on a consistent level that is non-threatening or neutral, the brain just shuts off—the ticking clock, the shoes on your feet, a necklace around your neck, the glasses on your face. The things that are consistently present, non-threatening, the mind shuts out.

Here is the important question: Why is it that yogis and Zen masters across different traditions show the same capacity to go past the habituation response? Why would one seeking enlightenment need to go past that profound level of conditioning of the mind-brain system? If you think about it, whenever we talk about what the highest is—whether it's bodhicitta, Buddha mind, Christ consciousness, the Divine Self, Unity Consciousness, or any of these descriptions of the highest consciousness—it always includes that It is present at all times, in all places. If you have a mechanism in your brain that automatically tunes out what is always present, it is a closed door that is always going to prevent you from knowing at all times and all places the living presence of the Divine. Mystics of all traditions develop a capacity of consciousness to go past this brain gate and then report living in the ever-present Light of the Infinite.

Our consciousness learns through the foundational practices to leave behind these mind-brain mechanisms so that we can be continuously aware of what is continuously present, the Infinite, which of course is not only non-threatening, but boundlessly loving, boundlessly compassionate, boundlessly awake—that is our nature. We have to be able to go far past that fundamental level of mind-brain conditioning that is constantly in survival mode. The foundational practices of mindfulness, mantra meditation, and Witness Consciousness help us develop that capacity. It's not enough to have peak experiences or flashy visions; these are ephemeral.

Mindfulness

The practice of mindfulness is essential for stabilizing attention and awareness, while creating greater freedom and detachment from the ego mind. If you imagine the night sky, expansive and clear, with a spotlight shining into the sky, illuminating whatever it shines on, you'll get a sense of awareness and attention. Within the broad sky of awareness, attention is the spotlight we use to focus consciousness on a narrow field in the broad sky. Mindfulness practices involve holding your attention steady on one thing, say the breath, while in a relaxed state, watching with detached dispassion whatever arises, as all the stuff of the mind arises and subsides in the sky of awareness. Thoughts, feelings, sensations, memories, fantasies about the future or the past come and go. You can do this right now.

MINDFULNESS EXERCISE

Take a moment to settle your body into a comfortable upright sitting posture as you would for meditation, allow your breath to slow and deepen while inviting all the muscles in your body to soften and warm. All tension can melt away from the body as you feel the gentle heaviness of your legs resting at ease, your body resting at ease, your arms and hands resting comfortably as your neck and shoulders soften and let go as well. Even the muscles in your scalp and face can soften, warm and let go. There's nothing to do except follow the breath all the way as it comes in and all the way as it goes out. Focus your attention on sensations of the breath flowing in and out through your nose, along with the sensation of the rise and fall of your diaphragm. Remain mindful of those two areas, nose and abdomen, during the entire length of the breath coming in and going out. When your attention wanders to something else, immediately bring it back to the flow of the breath. You might start with setting a timer for ten minutes and work your way up to forty-five minutes of engaging in this profound and powerful practice.

Do this mindfulness practice daily for forty-five minutes and in just three weeks you will have begun to change your brain, as well as free your mind! Mindfulness isn't limited to breath awareness. That is an initial exercise that one does for years, and then it becomes natural and effortless. Over time the practice of mindfulness expands to being continuously aware and mindful of states of lovingkindness and boundless compassion, with insight into what arises that blocks those states and what brings them back to awareness. In this way, you are keeping the ordinary ego mind in its proper role and cultivating the greater field for full awakening to flower.

Mantra

We've spoken about mantra many times so far in this book. The Shiva Sutras say that mantra is the basis of mind; it is the basis of the subtle body and the physical body; it is a living throb, a pulse of Shakti Kundalini that you are given to remove the veils of ignorance separating you from the truth of your sublime nature. It has the power to totally transform the mind and body, awaken Kundalini and nurture it to complete its unfolding. Mantra meditation is an essential practice, though it can be engaged on different levels. The throb of the awareness of pure "I Am," of bare awareness of unbounded Consciousness is the heart of mantra. Whether one is immersed in that or immersed in repeating Om Namah Shivaya, it is all the same to Kundalini. At the end of chapter 3 is a mantra meditation practice for you to enjoy. Mantra japa, the practice of repeating the mantra is done for meditation as well as throughout the day. Returning the mind over and over again to its source, through mantra, frees the mind from the patterns of thinking and reacting that it normally engages in. When used in meditation you can completely dissolve the mind in mantra. When used while carrying on your everyday activities, it works to retrain the mind, keep it focused and free it from old habit patterns. Mantra is a very potent practice for cultivating Kundalini awakening and unfolding. We'll study it further in chapter 11.

Witness Consciousness

Witness Consciousness expands mindfulness to watching all experience from the place of the Witness, the transcendent one, Shakti/Shiva, who watches all with boundless love for its Self as its Self. In Witness Consciousness meditation, you gradually let go of the ego mind, the little self, and merge with the Infinite Self, the Witness of all the states of consciousness. You move from being the seen, the object of perception, to being the Seer, the one who is never an object of perception. I discussed this in chapter 5 and a meditation practice for moving into Witness Consciousness is at the end of that chapter.

The simple clear light of awareness, pure unbounded Consciousness, without even a sense of "being" defining it, is your nature; this is where your freedom lies. That unbounded awareness is known in silence, in stillness. That's the stillness against which all the movements of the mind are perceived, whether those movements are thoughts or feelings, memories or images, intuitions or realizations—they all rest on that stillness, that expansiveness of pure awareness. We can dial in to that; we can open our consciousness to that awareness which is the throb of Shakti; that's the throb of Kundalini illuminating all that is. She is that light of awareness that allows us to perceive whatever the thoughts, the images, the sensations, the feelings might be. That Self-luminous, pure awareness is Shakti, the Witness of all. She becomes the mantra Om Namah Shivaya; that too is a throb, a vibration of Shakti, and carries with it that same power to cut through the mind and bring us to the direct experience of who and what we are beyond the mind. At the same time Shakti, Witness Consciousness, illumines the process of becoming the ego, the ordinary mind.

We know what it is to experience the world from that contracted awareness of the ordinary mind, from the awareness of identification with this form, but Kundalini Shakti is inviting us to know the expansiveness of being all forms as well as our own form, with the illuminated awareness that is free to watch from a place of sublime ecstasy and peace. In the process of Kundalini expanding our awareness, She also makes us aware of how we become the limited forms of our own creation, how we take on identities. Kundalini illuminates quite vividly how our mind is doing that moment by moment. Thoughts create reality; we become what we are through the mind's power acting moment by moment.

One time a wise saint was about to go on a journey with his disciple and before they were leaving the saint said to the young man, "No matter what, don't become anything," and his disciple looked at him quizzically, not really understanding what the old saint was talking about, but knew that masters sometimes talked in ways that you didn't necessarily understand. And the master said again, "Remember, don't become anything." As they journeyed on through the day, going deeper and deeper into the forest, day became evening, and they needed to find a place to stay overnight. They came upon what looked like one of the king's palaces, deep in the forest, but nobody was there. The king must have been away and they thought, "Well, we could stay there and spend the night." They entered the palace and fell asleep. Sometime in the early morning, some of the palace guards began to return. It turned out that this in fact was a hunting lodge for the king when he was out in the forest. As the guards came to prepare the dwelling for the king's arrival, they found these two sleeping in one of the rooms in the king's palace. First they went to the old man and asked, "Who are you? What are you doing here?" The old man just looked at them and didn't answer, didn't say anything and the guard said, "Oh, he's just and old man, we don't know what's going on with him," and they carried him out and set him aside under a tree outside.

The disciple awakening and seeing the guards handle his guru, his master, in this way, became really angry and furious. He started to yell to the guards, "Don't you know who he is? He's the great master, he's my guru—you can't handle him like that! Who do you think you are?" Immediately the guards turned to the young man and said, "Who do you think you are? Who are you to be in the king's palace?" and they grabbed him, beat him, and threw him down the hill where he landed at the feet of his master. There sat the master; there was the disciple beat up and bruised and as the disciple gathered himself and looked at the master, all the master could say was, "What did you become?" In that encounter with the guards the disciple had become a number of things. He'd become the indignant disciple, he'd become the angry person, he'd become the defender of his teacher, and he'd become one thing after another, all of which led to the kind of abuse and treatment that he received. Whereas the master, who became nothing, was treated like nothing; he was just taken outside and left under a tree.

We have to watch moment by moment what we become. What have you become right now as you watch your thoughts? What did you become when you first woke up in the morning? What will you become five minutes from now? What will you become over lunch or at the next meeting? Moment by moment our mind is becoming one thing after another. Each thought, each feeling has with it an identity that we become, that we inhabit and then experience the consequences having become it. Part of what Shakti illumines is that process of becoming, how we become one thing after another after another.

Shakti gives us the power to step back and let go of that process. She also empowers us to choose consciously what to become in this moment. That's the kind of freedom that awakened Kundalini gives us, the freedom to see how we become things, to step back and truly see. What did I become with my wife, what did I become with my child, what did I become at work, what did I become when I saw that person who intimidates me, what did I become with that person I thought was inferior? We're constantly becoming. We can see that some of the things that we've become serve no purpose, or they serve ignorance, or they serve anger, they serve fear, or they just create painful ways of being and interacting in our life. They don't serve our sublime nature; they don't serve our being wise and compassionate, being patient and kind. So we have to let go of the old forms that no longer serve, let them go over and over again, dissolving them with the great Shakti of mantra that releases the bound energy the matrika shaktis created. Cleared of those limiting forms, we come back to the truth of who and what we are, knowing what our choices are and where our freedom lies.

Coming into that state of freedom, into the boundless joy and illumination of our true nature, isn't a matter of just doing that while our eyes are closed, or only when we're in the midst of a beautiful chant, or we're in a beautiful temple, or a great meditation hall, or a lovely place in nature. Those are good places to start, but that power and that experience are available at all times and all places and can visit us at any time, inviting us to merge in the state of steady wisdom, continuous knowing.

One morning the Devi said to me in my internal awareness, in my mind:

> This is it, my Friend!
> This day is it!
> This day is the unfolding
> of the glory of God!
> This is it, my Friend!
> This hour is it!
> This hour is the unfolding
> of the glory of God!
> This is it, my Friend!
> This breath is it!
> This breath is the unfolding
> of the glory of God!
> This is it, my Friend!
> This creation is it!
> This creation is the unfolding
> of the glory of God!
>
> KALIDAS[1]

I saw and felt that what She was saying was absolutely true. I was ecstatic; tears rolled down my cheeks! But as I looked around, of course I also saw that I was in my car, stuck in rush hour traffic, heading into the hospital in Cincinnati at the beginning of my workday. I noticed how my body was feeling. I was just a few days from going in for the first of two surgeries I was about to have for a back injury, which was causing considerable pain. None of these things diminished the ecstatic feeling in the least, nor did I feel separate from the whole wonderful fabric of reality in the moment. It's in the midst of this or any context that the unfolding of the glory of God and the full experience of that reality is present. That's what's available to us by the grace of Shakti Kundalini, that's what She wants to give us.

That's what we cultivate, the openness to receive, that expanded awareness. It's only the mind that blocks that full awareness; unbounded awareness is always present. When we've cultivated that expansiveness and received the grace of Shakti, then that awareness blossoms in all kinds of situations. This expansive awareness is our essential nature and it's known in all traditions. There was a great Zen master who wrote, "Your body is not bounded by the surface of your skin, you know. The sun and the moon are your body. The oceans and rivers are your body. The whole universe is your body. The Buddha based his religion upon this mind, this consciousness, sometimes you call it 'one body,' sometimes you call it 'God,' we don't use that name for it, but when you observe that your mind is as boundless as the sky, an endless universe and your present state, this moment is here, that is all. All the teachings are in your heart, they are inherent, the intrinsic law of your nature. You cannot find this anywhere outside of yourself."[2]

OVERCOMING THE MIND'S ATTACHMENT TO MOVEMENT

The foundational practices seem so simple—stay present with the mind, just witnessing and watching it; stay present with the mantra and mindful of that inner sound repeating itself over and over. To the ordinary mind, these are so simple and repetitive that it often dismisses their power and importance. The mind thinks, "No, not this same old boring exercise! Give me something that's, you know, full of light and color, sound and movement!" In part, it's because the ordinary mind is addicted to movement; it loves to be stimulated by movement. Working with the ego mind to cultivate the field of awareness for awakening involves training the mind to rest in stillness.

Research shows that if you put a person in a sensory deprivation tank where there's no visual stimuli, no auditory stimuli, where they're floating and the water is the exact temperature of the body, so everything seems exactly the same and there's no sensory information coming in, the mind can't stand it. Within minutes they will start to hallucinate. The mind literally starts creating sounds and feelings and visuals, because it is so addicted to movement. Kundalini Shakti and the practices take us beyond that by immersing us in profound stillness. Kundalini draws us into levels of absolute stillness where the mind doesn't move at all, but we can become more awake, knowing that in that profound stillness there's a whole other quality of awareness. There's a whole other dimension of clear, awake awareness that isn't conditioned by the limitations of the ordinary mind, the ego mind, the waking state, the dream state, or ultimately even the deep sleep state. Kundalini immerses you in this deepest state of meditation, the state of turiya.

TRANSCEND AND INCLUDE THE EGO

Kundalini's extraordinary transformative process doesn't turn the ego mind into the Self, or Buddha; ego doesn't become your essential, Infinite Universal Consciousness—the ego mind gets transformed into a strong, creative, sensitive, intuitive, enthusiastic, compassionate servant. It doesn't get destroyed in the way that most people understand the concept of ego destruction at the outset of spiritual practice. The ego isn't the enemy, and we don't have to make it an adversary. Kundalini created the ego mind along with the body, brain, and everything else. We have to develop the discrimination to perceive its highest purpose. The ego isn't destroyed; it is our sole identification with the ego mind that is destroyed, bondage to the mind-body construct is destroyed, but they continue to exist. We need a conventional self based on the mind-body complex. Without the ego mind we couldn't function in the world, we would be psychotic.

The ego mind becomes transformed into a skillful servant, being able to act in a way that makes it ever at the service of what your highest nature is and continuously informed by your Self. In many ways sadhana makes the ego mind stronger and more skillful than it was before doing such practices. Sadhana practices support us being focused and skillful in the world as well as going beyond the world—transcend and include. Sadhana practices reduce the ego mind's grip on consciousness and allow us to become aware of the higher impulses from the Self that can redirect the ego mind. You gain the freedom to be detached from ego and have your true Self inform it with boundless wisdom, compassion, love, and kindness. Then the ordinary mind develops toward manifesting these qualities in our everyday actions. This is the sacred dharma of the ego: to function within the bounds of serving the highest good, the Divine Within, your boundlessly compassionate Buddha/Christ/Infinite nature.

Once there was an extraordinarily creative master woodworker, a true artisan, using his skills for building, carving, molding wood in marvelous ways. But he fell, hit his head and forgot who he was. He thought he was just his hands. He became completely focused and obsessed with his hands to the point where he neglected everything else about himself because all that had dropped out of his awareness. (There are forms of brain damage where people neglect half their body because they don't recognize it as part of themselves!) People cared deeply for him and couldn't figure out how to get him back. One person even suggested cutting off his hands to force him to come back to himself. What a horrible approach! Instead, his loved ones touched his body lovingly, touched his face, caressed his shoulders, massaged his back and legs and feet, and in this loving manner they were inviting his mind, his feelings, and his awareness to connect with all that he was. Gradually he reconnected with his wholeness.

Just because we've become identified solely with this tiny part of ourselves, the ego mind, the organ for grasping and doing in this world, doesn't mean we should cut it off in order to regain the awareness of our true expansive nature. Language about cutting off the ego, cutting off the head of the ego, and killing the ego permeates spiritual literature and has led many people astray, binding people to an inner war, making people engage in self-mutilation, self-flagellation, and terrible things. We don't have to cut off the ego any more than the woodworker needed to have his hands cut off. We have to go beyond the confines of the ego mind and allow consciousness to regain its awareness of the fullness of the Self, even as the ego mind continues to function, but now as a faithful and dedicated servant of the Divine. The ego mind has to be reminded of its boundaries and then it can function properly within its own skin.

Kundalini cuts the root of ego's delusion of Self-concealment, which allows for the Infinite to identify with the finite. The finite isn't destroyed in order to regain access to the boundless awareness that already exists, the Unity Consciousness of the Self. Kundalini awakens us to the full experience of knowing that the Infinite transcends and subsumes all the finite worlds in the waking, dream, and deep sleep states. Only She can give that gift. Self-effort can take one all the way up to the ajna chakra, but to go beyond, to pass through the knot of the causal body, requires the command, the grace of Shakti. She may grant you a temporary visitor's visa from time to time and allow you in, but one has to be Her or Shiva to know that transcendent realm as home!

SEVA

Seva is selfless service. This is a practice of central importance in sadhana and particularly in Kundalini sadhana because it helps to integrate into everyday life the transformations that Kundalini produces. You can be inspired by meditative experiences of oneness, of seeing the divinity of others, and then in the crucible of seva that vision is integrated into action. By offering selfless service, the ego mind learns to put aside all concern for itself, its comfort, its status, and its rewards to become absorbed in simply serving others. The ego mind is transformed, and you further cultivate the awareness of being more than just the ego mind, awake to the fullness of who you are and who you serve. Conscious parenting is one of the greatest arenas for sadhana and seva. Lovingly and mindfully serving the beings we're entrusted with as our children is one of the most sacred endeavors we can engage in.

> "It is critical to serve others, to contribute actively to others' well-being. I often tell practitioners that they should adopt the following principle: regarding one's own personal needs, there should be as little involvement or obligation as possible. But regarding service to others, there should be as many possible involvements and obligations as possible. This should be the ideal of a spiritual person."
>
> HIS HOLINESS THE DALAI LAMA[3]

Seva is an easy practice to do and a very difficult practice to master. It is an essential practice for retraining the ego mind. We can mindfully bring the attitude of selfless service to caring for loved ones, doing our work, fulfilling our dharma, even offering up our practices in the service of all. However, the ego has its ways of infiltrating this practice, distracting one in the midst of the practice with a running commentary in the moment that is full of judgment, keeping its agenda for recognition or reward operating in the background, or ambitiously trying to outdo others in their selfless service! The ego is very creative! We can laugh at its antics and bring it back to the practice of selflessly serving. There's an old text in the Christian tradition by Brother Lawrence called *The Practice of the Presence of God*, which is a beautiful and inspiring book on seva and mindfulness combined.

Dedicated practices of seva outside of home and work are important. By serving youth, serving disadvantaged people, serving the environment, or any of the countless ways of offering dedicated service for which there is no seeking of rewards, there is no chance for the ego mind to hold an agenda of getting noticed at work or getting something from family members. It is simply your offering of selfless service. If you are used to being in charge at work, it can be good to teach the ego surrender and humility through serving in a way where you're not in charge.

When I was managing an ashram in Philadelphia for Baba and Gurumayi, one of the main practices was seva, as it was in all the ashrams. It was so moving to see people who were from all different backgrounds, all different levels of wealth and education, come together and offer seva by doing everything from cleaning toilets to running the kitchen or helping with financial aspects of running the organization. It was also a powerful practice for wearing off the rough edges of the egos involved!

FOOD AND EXERCISE

Cultivating physical and mental health and resilience helps create the optimal conditions for awakening and unfolding Kundalini. It's not that we have to be in ideal health mentally and physically for Kundalini to awaken and evolve, but taking care of the mind-body vehicle in ways that best support our wellbeing decreases what Kundalini has to transmute or overcome in the process of unfolding. This is also another area in which the ego mind is deconditioned and engaged in relating to the vehicles of mind and body in new, healthier ways.

There are so many layers of cultural and familial conditioning that impact how a person views their body and mind, treats their body and mind, and identifies with them. All of these are transformed through awakening. Becoming aware and mindful of this conditioning empowers you to step back from it and, from a more expanded, detached, and compassionate consciousness, treat the mind and body with informed and caring attention.

As Shakti moves through the mind and body it heightens people's awareness of various aspects of these vehicles. Watch how your diet affects your energy and how it affects your mind's state. Kundalini sadhana demands that we become very sensitive to understanding how Shakti is guiding us in the moment. Do we need to follow a vegetarian diet, or do we need to supplement our diet in non-vegetarian ways? You'll notice that some foods give you greater energy and support your health while other foods diminish your energy, increase irritability, or douse you with feelings of heaviness and lethargy. Other foods might interfere with meditation, and you'll learn to notice that. The process of Kundalini unfolding requires deepening discrimination as you discern what Shakti is telling you about the marvelous workings of the energy system that we call the body and mind. Increased awareness and freedom from all the layers of conditioning allow the ego mind to best serve the needs of your mind and body as Kundalini transforms them. With meditation our awareness becomes more and more refined and subtle, able to follow the promptings, the call of Shakti, including the answers to the questions: What am I going to eat for lunch? What am I going to drink? What foods am I attracted to and why? What foods am I averse to? It's not as simple as following a dietary regimen, Shakti's much more subtle than that. Food needs to be fresh and full of prana. Until you feel clear about discerning how Shakti is shaping your diet, it is good to follow a healthy, balanced vegetarian diet.

I remember Baba saying, "If you don't feed the Shakti, the Shakti will eat you alive." In Kundalini sadhana you have to develop the discrimination to know how to feed Shakti so that it makes your body bright and luminous, healthy and full. There are times when Shakti is very active and people need to eat rich foods including butter, dairy, and sweets. I went through a period where Kundalini's fire was so intense that my ordinary vegetarian diet couldn't keep up with it. My body became emaciated-looking. I had to eat more rich dairy foods. Then after a year or so it shifted again. Some people need to eat fish, poultry, or meat for periods of time. Some people become aware of food allergies they didn't know they had because their mind wasn't sensitive enough to discern the impact of what they were eating on their mental and physical well-being. Whatever one is eating, it needs to be fresh, free of toxins and chemicals, and include foods with a great deal of prana—fresh fruits and vegetables. Root crops, potatoes, carrots, beets, yams, and the like can be grounding when that is needed to help balance and stabilize the mind. I've worked with numerous people who found it helpful to consult a nutritionist to become more discerning about their food.

It's also important to look at how we feed the mind because that's another way that we feed Shakti. What do we engage the mind in? What do we pay attention to? What are we contemplating? What are we reading, what are we watching? What kind of company do we keep in the mind? These too feed Shakti or diminish Shakti. Exercise your discrimination that develops from following the call of Shakti, as subtle as it may be, and discover what makes you feel brighter, clearer, more alive, full of energy, more compassionate, steadier. Follow the inner guidance of Shakti that leads you in the right directions.

It's the same with exercise. Explore and learn for yourself which types of exercise build your Shakti. One of the reasons why Kundalini awakening was sought after by yogis was because of how Shakti guides yoga practices. There are eighty-four thousand *asanas* (yoga "postures") of which eighty-four are said to be central. In the ordinary practice of hatha yoga, you would learn from somebody and go through a routine of numerous hatha yoga postures. It would take many years to master them. But you might be learning postures that aren't necessarily what your body and subtle body need. Awakened Kundalini draws you to the postures that you need to be doing. With awakened Kundalini the practice of asanas goes from being a set of postures that's being dictated by the ego mind, to following the promptings of awakened Kundalini directing you to what is best for you. It may not even be an asana or a pranayama that's written down somewhere, but your body and prana are going to change in ways that are exactly what you need because it is directed by Kundalini. The transcendent intelligence of Shakti is now guiding that process, and it will relieve even ordinary yoga processes from being solely ego directed. This is the difference between "my will be done" and "thy will be done." Even in the domain of exercise, you can be attuned to the level of energy, the clarity, the presence of Shakti in your body and in your mind. Let that guide you in what you're doing. Most people who are physically capable of it benefit from incorporating aerobic exercise in their weekly practices. The increased cardiovascular activity and breathing are great for clearing and circulating prana. Regularly being out in nature is balancing and grounding for your energy as well. Daily or at least weekly outdoor activity can make a huge difference for supporting a more expansive and fluid state of mind and body.

The mind and body are the fields for awakening and unfolding Kundalini. They are sublime vehicles of consciousness for knowing and serving the truth of who you are, as well as everyone and all of creation. Practices—such as meditation, cultivating stillness, detaching from ego, seva, physical exercise, and consciously feeding the body and mind—can integrate awareness into every moment and de-condition the mind, body, and brain in ways that free you from ingrained patterns. By approaching the mind and body as a field for awakening, you can cultivate the body and mind so they are in the best state possible to serve and participate in the ecstasy of creation and the unfolding of Kundalini.

The greatest practice is Compassion,
The greatest discipline is Patience,
The greatest path is Love.
Resolve to faithfully and enthusiastically follow these,
And you will know yourself to be Free.

KALIDAS[4]

10

The Eight Limbs of Classical Yoga

The word *yoga* means "union" and refers to the Unity Consciousness that the seeker realizes through union with the Self, the Infinite. The word *yoga* also means "to yoke," as you would yoke horses to a wagon to pull it where you want it to go. Through yoga practices, you yoke the energies of prana, mind, senses, and body to direct them toward transformation and the direct experience of Unity Consciousness, the highest attainment possible for a human, the state of true freedom.

The yoga paradigm provides us with a deep understanding of the nature of Kundalini, how She creates the causal, subtle, and physical bodies, and how She binds consciousness to these vehicles to create the experience of finite existence, which we know so well. The yoga paradigm also maps out paths to freedom from bondage, ways created by Kundalini, which reflect her dynamic actions for cutting the knot of avidya, the primal ignorance that initiates the process of the Infinite becoming finite. There are numerous ancient forms of yoga, including mantra yoga, laya yoga, bhakti yoga, jnana yoga, hatha yoga, and raja yoga, which is also known as Ashtanga yoga or the Classical yoga of Patanjali.

Ashtanga means "eight limbs." These eight limbs of yoga described in the classic Yoga Sutras of Patanjali, written down approximately two thousand years ago from ancient oral teachings, instruct the aspirant studying with a master how to end bondage and suffering by reducing and finally extinguishing the vrittis, the thought waves that cloud our consciousness and obscure the ever-present and direct experience of the Self. The eight limbs are a comprehensive set of practices that also prepare the mind and body for Kundalini awakening. They give the seeker clear means for easing Kundalini's purifying flow through the subtle and physical bodies. The eight limbs are: yamas (5 restraints), niyamas (5 further restraints and observances), asana (postures, seat of awareness), pranayama (control of prana/breath), pratyahara (withdrawal of the senses from the outside world), dharana (focusing attention), dhyana (meditation), and samadhi (absorption in Unity Consciousness). By doing all the practices of the eight limbs of yoga, you develop the strength of the container—mind and body—to hold the enormous energies moved by Kundalini. I say *all* the practices because the ego mind likes to look at the list of practices as an à-la-carte menu—choosing asanas and pranayama, maybe some dharanas, based on what it feels like doing in the moment. Just like that, the ego mind takes over one's sadhana, perverting it to reinforce the ego's self-cherishing mode of existence. Prior to Kundalini awakening, one does all the practices as a comprehensive approach to cultivating the field for awakening. After Kundalini awakening, Shakti and your teacher will guide you on the right balance of practices for your sadhana.

The yoga practices given by Kundalini, the mother of all yogas, are extremely helpful as supports for the process of Kundalini unfolding. The esoteric goal of all yogas has been the awakening of Kundalini, and once Kundalini is awakened, these practices support the graceful unfolding of the transformative power of Consciousness as it fashions anew the mind and body. Aspects of Ashtanga yoga and other forms of yoga often spontaneously arise for people after Kundalini awakening. For example, spontaneously hearing mantras arising within as in mantra yoga, or becoming absorbed in visions of light or divine sounds as in laya yoga, or being overwhelmed by love and devotion as in bhakti yoga.

The eight limbs of yoga begin with practices called the *yamas* and the *niyamas,* the restraints and the observances. These are the foundation of all the other practices. The yamas and niyamas are moral and ethical practices of self-restraint and self-regulation that inform all the other practices. They include attitudes, values, and ways of acting that are essential for guiding and focusing all our energies toward the goal of yoga and Kundalini unfolding. The yamas and niyamas are:

nonviolence, truthfulness, nonstealing, sexual continence, nongreed, purity of body and mind, contentment, austerity, scriptural study and constant remembrance of the Self, and surrender to the Divine. We'll look at them in more detail after I've described the other limbs, as they are a very important foundation for the other six limbs and are often a neglected set of practices.

ASANA

Asanas are the postures—the movement and flow aspects of yoga with which many people are familiar. They develop the body and mind in specific ways, and they can help with Kundalini processes because the postures are really psychophysical exercises that clear the body and mind of blocks and open energy channels for prana (one of the energies that Kundalini creates) to move more freely through them.

Too often I've encountered people who thought postures were all there was to yoga, as if it were just another exercise routine. Nothing could be further from the truth. *Yoga* means "union," union with the Divine, the Self. Asana practice is aimed at reducing the vrittis caused by the body and mind. If one makes the body strong, healthy, and able to sit comfortably, then when one sits in meditation the mind will not be disturbed by sensations, aches, and pains produced by the body. Asanas make the flow of prana steadier and more harmonious.

Asana also means "seat." The postures are intended to help one develop a seat, a meditation posture, which is necessary for the full practice of yoga. There is no yoga without meditation. Without meditation all you have is yoga exercise. A comfortable, erect meditative posture also facilitates the flow of prana and the eventual rising of Kundalini Shakti as it traverses up the sushumna nadi (the central energy channel of the subtle body), clearing the samskaras and transporting one's consciousness to higher levels.

Research on the positive effects of yoga asanas is building and shows them to benefit mind-body health in numerous ways ranging from lowering stress, cholesterol levels, and blood pressure to increasing focus, decreasing the severity and frequency of seizure disorders, improving sleep, and more. For our health-conscious culture, yoga asanas make perfect sense. They can lead people to discover the profound teachings that yoga offers as well. In Kundalini sadhana, asanas may occur spontaneously as Shakti moves one's body into postures. With awakened Kundalini, one has to be sensitive to the effects of postures. Use your discrimination to guide you in which postures to do, how intensely to do them, for how long, and when to stop or change the practice. Skilled guidance from a teacher familiar with awakened Kundalini, not just the concept of Kundalini, but awakened Kundalini, is important. This is true for all the practices.

PRANAYAMA

Pranayama is control of our breathing and the vital force, or prana, which is related to our breath and our mind. Prana is the subtle power linking matter and physical energy, on the one hand, with mind, consciousness, and subtle energies on the other. Regulating the prana influences our mind. Pranayama exercises are enormously powerful and shouldn't be practiced except under the guidance of a qualified teacher. For beginning meditation it's fine to simply allow the breath to flow spontaneously and naturally. As our breathing becomes rhythmic and natural, deeper and more diaphragmatic, the mind becomes quiet, the obscuring vrittis are further reduced. Silently and slowly repeating mantra in coordination with the breath, once on the inhalation and once on the exhalation, creates a natural pranayama that will completely absorb the mind. People frequently notice that pranayama happens spontaneously because of Kundalini awakening. Kriyas caused by Kundalini awakening often impact the breath, causing spontaneous retention of the breath—a form of kumbhaka pranayama, the slowing and deepening of the breath. Additional classic forms of this practice, like *bhastrika*, bellows breathing, also happen spontaneously due to Kundalini. People who have never done any yoga practices before regularly report these surprising events as part of their Kundalini experiences.

All the physical processes and practices up to this point have as their aim reducing the vrittis and empowering the yoga practitioner to begin the concentrative and meditative practices. One can just do yoga-style exercise, that's a very healthy choice. But in the practice of yoga, one understands that the yamas, niyamas, asanas, and pranayama all build toward and culminate in practices that bring one into samadhi, profound Unity Consciousness.

PRATYAHARA

The next limb, *pratyahara*, deals with withdrawing the mind from the senses and training the mind to be detached and aware, without following what the senses are usually calling the mind to attend to. A classic image of pratyahara is of the box turtle withdrawing its head and limbs inside its shell. In the same way, you pull your senses inside, leaving behind the outer world. This further reduces the obscuring thought waves and movements of the mind and body, moving them closer to Unity Consciousness and aligning them with Kundalini's unfolding.

DHARANA

Dharana, the sixth limb, is the focusing of the mind, the strengthening of the mind's ability to stay focused where you want it to be focused. It eliminates all the vrittis, the obscuring thought waves, caused by the senses in contact with the body and the outside world. Dharana is the practice of concentrating the flow of attention toward a single object within. The highest object of concentration is the Self or its vibratory equivalent, a mantra such as So'ham or Hamsa (Sanskrit for "I Am That"), Om Namah Shivaya, Om Kali Ma, Om Mani Padme Hum, or other empowered mantras. With the practice of mantra, as you focus entirely on the mantra, you dissolve the difference between the mantra, you as the repeater of the mantra, and the Divine as the source of the mantra. These are merged in the single awareness of pure "I Am," I am the mantra, I am the Infinite, I am Shakti, I am All-Embracing Loving Consciousness, I Am. Kundalini pulls the mind into this type of focused absorption and the next stages of meditation unfold spontaneously by her grace.

DHYANA

Dharana develops into the seventh limb, *dhyana,* or meditation—the uninterrupted flow of awareness toward the object of concentration as defined by Patanjali. Dhyana eliminates all remaining vrittis, thought waves, except the one of the object of concentration. The yoga practices described so far reduce the countless thought waves that usually occupy our minds down to just one. That one vritti might be the breath, the mantra, the Witness. Sometimes Kundalini will focus your entire awareness on inner sound, called *nada,* or visions of inner lights or overwhelming love. Whatever Kundalini is absorbing, your entire focus becomes a portal to the infinite. In Kundalini sadhana, meditation is of paramount importance. In the context of awakened Kundalini, meditation encompasses a broader range of processes than Patanjali's definition of meditation. The next chapter is devoted entirely to the transformative power of meditation in Kundalini sadhana.

SAMADHI

As the meditator eliminates the last remaining vritti, the practices culminate in *samadhi,* the eighth limb, where the subject-object split dissolves, all duality is gone leaving only Unity Consciousness. Sage Patanjali differentiates samadhi that still has the seed of the focus of absorption present (savikalpa samadhi) from the samadhi in which there isn't even the seed (nirvikalpa samadhi). Through empowered mantra, or directly through her power, Kundalini draws you into the unbounded awareness of being the very source of mantra, all sounds and words dissolve into the Infinite spaciousness of pure Being. Tat Twam Asi: Thou Art That.

However, to attain this state through the practice of yoga without awakened Kundalini one is warned: be prepared to pursue the perfection of each of those eight limbs over lifetimes. Awakened Kundalini gracefully brings about these states and supports the practitioner's ongoing self-effort to enter and stabilize these states.

YAMAS AND NIYAMAS

These two foundational sets of practices for yoga are often given very little atten- tion in the study and practice of yoga in the West. Millions of people go to yoga studios to practice. What that often means for them is that they're practicing postures, breathing exercises, relaxing in the corpse pose, and feeling good as a result. Yoga has been adopted in the West as a way to enhance and sustain one's health. That's a good goal and a good use of it, but it's also a very limited use of it—as wonderful as it is to be de-stressed and healthier, these are minimal side effects of what the practices of yoga are truly about. The practices of yoga are all aimed at giving us the experience of union with the Infinite and living from that intimate knowledge every moment of every day, being able to look at all beings with that same vision of their divinity, and seeing this as clearly as we see their human shortcomings. Just as the lofty goal of yoga is often overlooked, the practices of the yamas and the niyamas often get overlooked.

The yamas and niyamas help to ground and steady our mind and body. They're particularly important when Kundalini has been activated—a lot of people who feel like they're struggling with Kundalini awakening do so because the ego mind is challenged to contain and integrate transpersonal experiences and energies. The yamas and niyamas help develop an unshakeable foundation.

Yamas: Five Practices of "Not Doing"

Ahimsa: nonviolence. This is the first practice of the first limb of yoga and it forms the basis of one's entire sadhana, one's entire life. It's abstaining from any kind of violence, and that needs to be practiced internally as well. People begin to master it externally, they restrain themselves from being nasty or violent with another person, but the way they talk to themselves may be brutal, or even horribly violent. Ahimsa has to be practiced in relationship to oneself as well as others.

Satya: abstaining from lying. Most people think they are honest and avoid big lies, but the practice of abstaining from lying has subtleties. Think of all the ways the ego mind tries to tell itself little fibs to get through the day and pat itself on the back, or smooth over something it did wrong, or lay the blame off on somebody else. It means setting aside all those tendencies in order to simply be present, clear, and aware. It's that open awareness that allows us to be fully present and say, "Oh, no, that's not true. The truth is my mind did this, or my actions were that. I don't have to lie about it. I don't have to cover it up. I can be very clear and present with it." You are not your mind and body, but your conventional self is accountable for their actions and the consequences they create. Seeing the mind and body clearly and truthfully empowers you to be skillful in training and inspiring them to serve the Self. Sometimes the best expression of truth is what Buddha called noble silence! Say nothing that will bring harm. All these practices on one level strengthen the ego mind, but they strengthen it in service of something higher than itself and strengthen it to resist and halt the ordinary tendencies of the conditioned ego mind. New research even shows that there are health benefits to not lying! As if we needed research to prove that!

Asteya: abstaining from stealing. The gross form of stealing is easy for most of us to control; you're not going to rip off somebody's car—but the ego mind is, by its very nature as the power of self-appropriation, a thief! It appropriates to itself, or attempts to, everything it desires. You pull into a parking lot, and it has stolen that parking space; it has said, "That's my space." Well, who was it that laid claim to that parking space and then got angry that somebody else got their car into it first? Abstaining from stealing means becoming aware of and ceasing all the different ways that the ego mind is constantly appropriating things that don't belong to it. This includes qualities of your true nature, your true Self that the ego takes as its own. Consciousness doesn't belong to the ego mind;

Consciousness belongs to your true Self. The ego mind is like the moon, and the mind is often symbolized by the moon, because just as the moon only shines by reflected light, the limited consciousness of the mind is only a mere reflection of the luminous Divine Self. Restraining the mind's many forms of self-appropriation is asteya. Awakened Kundalini makes people very aware of the wanting and grasping nature of the ego mind that underlies the stealing. As Shakti repeatedly immerses your consciousness in the fullness of the Self those qualities are extinguished.

Brahmacharya: abstaining from sexual activity, which classically means celibacy, but is also applied by refraining from sexually acting out and being disciplined in one's sex life, restraining and harnessing the power of sexual desires. It is another facet of training the ego mind. When Kundalini is working on the second chakra, people can experience their sexual impulses extremely intensified or completely quieted or fluctuating. Being able to sustain the detached awareness necessary to simply watch the fluctuations of the energy and not be identified with them or driven by them is critically important.

Aparigraha: abstaining from possessiveness, from the clinging, attached behavior that is typical of the ego mind. This practice further detaches one from the ego and the cultural conditioning of consumerism, though all one has to do is look through a yoga magazine to see the ways that consumerism and spiritual materialism infiltrate the yoga exercise milieu. Awakened Kundalini often inspires people to simplify their lives. They find they don't need all the stuff they accumulated and donate their surplus to those in need.

Just by practicing the yamas, you begin to really contain and transform the ego mind and cultivate a detached, dispassionate awareness that empowers you to step back and look at the mind. This gives the ego mind the freedom to learn how to selflessly and sensitively serve your highest nature. The conscious disciplined practice of the yamas cultivates and makes fertile the field for awakening Kundalini. The five niyamas, the observances, take you even further in creating the optimal conditions for Kundalini awakening and unfolding.

Niyamas: The Five Observances

Saucha: observing purity, to act in ways that keep your body, mind, and environment, pure, clean, and uplifting. In the practice of yoga, one is dedicated to doing things that are uplifting, that reflect the knowledge that you are the Self, you are Buddha, as is everyone else. Wherever you are, wherever you go, welcome your true nature into that place, into this moment with purity and clarity.

Santosha: practicing contentment. This one often challenges people because we have a trillion dollar advertising industry that's determined to make you feel discontent so you will buy, buy, buy in hopes of finding happiness. Practicing contentment is another way that you're doing the hero's journey, stepping outside the confines of a society that wants to practice discontent, materialism, and consumerism. Instead, you're practicing contentment and simplicity. This practice empowers you to realize you don't have to wait for rare moments of contentment to enjoy the ease and peace that go with it. You cultivate santosha until it is your moment-by-moment experience. If we all did this one practice, we would save the environment, feed all the hungry, and have plenty of time left over to joyously love, dance, and create society anew!

Tapas: practicing austerity. Simplicity is at the heart of this niyama. It refers to the practice of letting go of all the extra things we clutter our life and mind with. It's leading a mindful life that isn't so austere that you have to run out to live in a barren cave, but it means watching what's going on with the ego mind and all its acquisitiveness, detaching and freeing oneself from that. It's living one's sadhana with discipline, which generates *tapasya,* heat, the fire of yoga. This arises from the friction that exists between the impulses of the ego mind heading off in all the conditioned pathways it usually follows, but now it is rubbing up against the practices—the yamas, niyamas, and other practices—that curb those impulses and direct your energy toward sadhana alone. These thwart the ego mind, and it can get quite heated in its reactions!

Tapasya is the inner transformative fire of yoga. The ego mind often balks at this fire! If something isn't pleasant or doesn't become pleasant fairly quickly, the ego mind looks for what is wrong, what needs to change to get back to a pleasurable experience. However, in sadhana, the displeasure of the ego mind can be exactly the signal that your efforts are on the right track if you are mindful of where that displeasure arises from. This means using your discrimination to discern what attachment is being confronted or what identification is being challenged that will lead to greater freedom. It's not pain for the sake of pain. If your hand has been clutching a rope for so long that it has gotten cramped in that position, it will hurt to pry your fingers off the rope. It will be painful to regain your full range of motion and flexibility.

So it is with the clinging, attached ego mind. Sometimes it is Kundalini that is prying the attached ego mind away from a person, situation, or possession that it needs to let go of to be free. These dynamics unfold spontaneously with Kundalini awakening.

Svadhyaya: self study. This includes study of scriptures, contemplative practices, and chanting practices. It's turning your attention toward things that are going to expand your understanding of sadhana, of your true nature, and the true nature of the Infinite, the Self. The more grounded one becomes in the knowledge and experience of the Self, bodhicitta, Christ consciousness, and the like, the easier it is to be detached and compassionate with the ego mind. The locus of one's identity gradually shifts as sadhana progresses.

· *Ishvara pranidhana:* the practice of surrendering to the Infinite, the Divine, in whatever form you like. The ego mind consciously engages in the practice of surrender, it isn't necessarily automatic or natural for it to do so at the outset of sadhana. Different traditions engage in this practice in varying ways. In the Tibetan Buddhist tradition, one might practice this by making vows to do literally millions of prostrations, physical full prostrations on the ground over and over and over again regardless of what this does to one's hands and knees. There are deep grooves worn in the stone floors of temples from Buddhist practitioners doing prostrations for centuries. A full *pranam,* or prostration, is a profound posture of surrender and devotion. It works powerfully to restructure the ego mind, bringing it into right relationship with the Infinitude of one's true nature—whether that's your Buddha nature exemplified by Guru Rinpoche, your personal guru, Tara, Kwan Yin, or Shiva/Shakti as Self, Jesus, Universal Consciousness, Love, or whatever you like to call it. That's what you're practice of surrender is aimed at, surrender to your own sublime boundlessly loving nature.

From this brief discussion of the yamas and niyamas, just the first two limbs of yoga, you can see that they are aimed at completely restructuring the ego mind. Many people find these practices happening spontaneously by Kundalini's impetus after awakening. People share with me how addictions fell away or how they began feeling like they wanted to give away so many of the things they had accumulated but didn't really need. They simplified their lives. Others found anger and irritability waning as their ability to step back and watch the mind from a place of contented ease grew stronger. If Kundalini hasn't yet awakened, then these practices cultivate the field and plant the seed of that awakening. Dedicated practice of the yamas and niyamas along with the other six limbs of classical yoga will eventually bring awakening. Studying with an accomplished teacher is essential in order to learn how to engage in the practices skillfully.

THE EIGHT LIMBS IN ONE PRACTICE

Meditation is the essential yoga practice, and it embodies all eight limbs. The yamas and niyamas are embodied in the preparation you do to sit for meditation. Take your seat and settle into your meditation posture. Your seat is your asana, your posture of meditation, which is both a physical posture as well as an inner posture of awareness. Allow your breath to slow and deepen as it becomes regular, smooth, and steady. This is your pranayama. Pull your attention within, letting go of all interest in the outer world as pratyahara deepens. Focus your mind on Om Namah Shivaya, Om Namah Shivaya, Om Namah Shivaya. Inwardly hear every sound of each syllable arising from the depths of consciousness and dissolving into silence. Become one-pointed in your concentration as dharana develops into dhyana. Om Namah Shivaya, Om Namah Shivaya, Om Namah Shivaya alone pervades your awareness. The mind and all sense of self merge with Om Namah Shivaya. The Om Namah Shivaya dissolves into the Infinite One—samadhi unfolds by the grace of Kundalini Shakti.

11

Meditation

Unfolding Kundalini's Grace

K undalini engages all the yogic practices and processes of purification and refinement of body and mind. These can happen
spontaneously with Kundalini sadhana and draw one into sublime states of meditation that the ego mind can't produce on its
own. As this happens repeatedly for months, years, or lifetimes,
one can eventually become steady in living samadhi, attaining continuous
samadhi, sahaja samadhi. Living samadhi means it's not just confined to when
you're sitting still or quiet with your eyes closed. It is a samadhi that is the
fourth state of consciousness, the turiya state of meditation—a state that is
always present and we learn to access it any time, any place. This is the highest
state that then informs the ordinary mind and infuses it with the boundless
love, ecstasy, and the all-embracing compassion of your sublime Self. This is the
goal of Kundalini unfolding. This is your true nature.

In this state we can be awake meditatively and see the mind and body in
deep sleep, dreaming, or waking state activities. But now the ego mind is carrying them out with the discipline of having done the practices that allow it to
be focused solely on serving your highest nature. In this way, turiya, the state
of the Infinite, informs the ego mind with its all-pervasive awareness—which
is Shakti—while leaving the ego mind intact, but completely transformed.

This highest state of living samadhi is already fully developed, fully present. Our consciousness is so bound through identification and attachment to the mind-body self that we only experience the narrow confines of that small container. Kundalini liberates our awareness from that container bestowing radical freedom even while transforming the mind-body self and increasing its relative freedom.

The practice of meditation for people with awakened Kundalini is one of following Shakti, surrendering to Her in the moment, as one sits with the intention to meditate, dissolving the mind in mantra or the source of mantra—pure I-awareness. Kundalini meditation is whatever Kundalini gives you as you sit with Her, delight in her mantra form, in her bare awareness, her pure Consciousness.

HAMSA MEDITATION EXERCISE

Start by sitting in a comfortable, erect meditation posture (unless the body needs support or to lie flat), allowing the breath to slow and deepen, becoming absorbed in the silent repetition of Hamsa (pure I-am awareness), *Ham* (Hummm…) as the breath comes in and *Sa* (Saaa…) as the breath goes out and witnessing what unfolds until the timer goes off ending that meditation period.

Hamsa invokes the awareness beyond words of "I am the Infinite, I am Shiva, I am the source, I Am." Repeating the mantra in synchrony with the breath invites the mind and body to settle more and more deeply. Taking refuge in the mantra and the breath, dissolving all thoughts in the mantra, calms the mind and body. Continuously bring the mind back to the silent repetition of the mantra until even the silent words of mantra dissolve into stillness. Physical movements or swaying may occur or other phenomena may come and go, while you remain the Witness, detached and aware, infinite and free, the mind returning over and over to the inner throb of the mantra. The mantra may change forms, dissolve all forms into spacious, bare awareness . . . the Witness, Seeing but never seen . . . the Self, within whom the universe is but a grain of sand. You'll find complete rest there.

THE WAY TO PEACE

Take refuge in your breath,
Let go of the mind and rest in the breath.
Like the very dearest of friends,
Your breath has accompanied you
    through all the pains, sorrows and joys of your life.
Take refuge in your breath,
With loving attention follow its every movement,
Unravel the mystery of where the breath
    finds repose.
Listen with rapt attention to your dear friend,
The breath has been speaking to you
    since you were born,
Discover the mantra it whispers to you continuously,
Affirming the infinitude of your Being,
HAMSA is the ground on which this mad dance
    of existence pounds on….
Unravel the mystery of where mantra arises,
    and where it dissolves.
Abide in Stillness—
    the refuge of the breath,
    the source of mantra,
    the womb of all,
    where form and emptiness embrace,
    where Truth alone is revealed.
    where Love dissolves the illusion
      of differences.

              KALIDAS[1]

Meditation purifies consciousness of the automatic tendency to identify with the mind and its content. In Kundalini sadhana, there are times when it's necessary to negate the attachment and identification with things that fill the mind because that bondage is creating pain and delusion. The mind may be clinging to an identity that is part of a relationship, a job, a dream, or an aspiration. Shakti often spontaneously brings the awareness in meditation of *neti, neti,* I'm not that, and I'm not that, and I'm not this other thing I've always identified with—freeing consciousness from the clutches of avidya and the conditioned mind. At other times, our mind may have become too divorced, renouncing the world in a way that disconnects us from the ecstatic living presence of the Divine. The ego mind turns against the world in its attempt to posture freedom, only to reveal its shallow disdain, not true renunciation. Shakti Kundalini may spontaneously bring up the awareness of *iti, iti,* I am this, and this and this, this body, this mind, this seat, this world, this universe, behold the wonder, the beauty, the sublime nature of this, and this and this; it's all Shiva, it's all Shakti, it's all Self! This awareness fills your mind! Love and bliss return! Follow Kundalini in meditation and receive all her gifts!

Kundalini meditation unfolds by Shakti's will, each time we sit, day after day, as the years and decades go by. The ego mind does the little things like making sure you've set aside time every day for meditation; it remembers to shut off your phone; it maintains the purity and simplicity of your meditation space; it practices sitting still without being rigid; it focuses its attention on the throb of Kundalini that is mantra. The ego mind is the servant, the housekeeper following the owner's orders. Kundalini is the owner and ruler of the house. She does everything of importance. The ego mind raises the sail, while the winds of grace move your vessel forward. Invoke Her with reverence, approach Her with devotion, and surrender to Her loving power. It will take you exactly where you need to go. You are the Infinite. That is your ultimate destination. She may take you on the scenic route to getting there. Be patient, She knows best.

Whatever arises, restrain the mind from getting attached to it or seeking to duplicate it. Each moment, each experience comes as a gift of Shakti. While it's there, one delights in that gift, and then the Shakti might completely drop it and move on, and something else replaces it. You will go through periods where meditation is just the ordinary mind being Witnessed as you're stepping back and letting go and stepping back and letting go. All this is the play of what unfolds in the sadhana of Kundalini awakening, and it's moving your consciousness toward that radical freedom that lies at your essence already.

Kundalini sadhana is classified as a tantric tradition. The word *tantra* in its earliest uses thousands of years ago in the Vedas was related to weaving. Tantra practices reveal the Divine woven into the fabric of every moment.

The approach of tantra embraces all of life and every moment as the time to know the Infinite. There is nothing that is not Shiva; there is nothing that is not Shakti! This attitude of fully embracing all of creation is part of what tantra conveys. Iti, Iti—and this, and this—is the all-inclusive way of tantra that expands sadhana to embrace every moment and every activity to realize that everything is Shiva, everything is Shakti, everything is your sublime Self. Every moment is pregnant with full Consciousness, with nirvana, with samadhi, with ecstasy.

As I mentioned earlier, even a sneeze can launch one into samadhi when approached as a tantric practice. But it requires extraordinary discipline and discrimination to practice tantra skillfully. These have to be developed first. In order to be able to leap into the Infinite off the springboard of a pleasure or delight, or even mind-stopping horror, tantra recognizes all these as leaping off points, but to make that leap in the moment demands the ability to instantaneously let go of the finite to merge with the Divine. My experience is that Kundalini Shakti bestows this quite effortlessly if the individual's sadhana requires it. In Kundalini sadhana, She determines what is needed, what isn't, and when. Everything else is the ego mind pursuing its same old agenda, but now spiritualized in the name of tantra.

Meditation is the crucible for transformation. Kundalini pulls you into meditation if you allow yourself to feel her embrace. Meditation frees you from lifetimes of karmas. It purifies the subtle body, the mind, and the physical body. It heals illnesses and cures you of the disease of ignorance. Meditation cuts all the illusory bonds limiting your consciousness to the ego mind and body. Meditation opens the heart to love beyond measure, beyond comprehension, beyond even imagination. You are a living, breathing expression of that love. You are a direct conduit to the ocean of love that is the Divine; let it pour forth into your world. Knowing this unfolds in meditation. Wisdom, profound insights, and realization all arise by Shakti's grace in meditation. Selflessness and unaffected humility emerge out of meditation. Become drunk on the wine of meditation, and live your life in wonder!

Kundalini delights in movement as much as in stillness. While meditating you might find your body gently rocking or swaying to the currents of Shakti flowing through it. Here is an exercise for tuning into the subtle movements of Kundalini.

SPIRAL MEDITATION

Sit comfortably upright in a good meditation posture. It can be on the floor or in a chair. Begin as you usually would by allowing the body and mind to settle, allowing your breathing to slow and deepen, while your mind and attention let go of the outside world and rest inside. Feel your torso and the column of space that runs from the base of your pelvis, up through the center of your body, up through your neck to the center of the top of your head. You might experience it as a column of light or the trunk of a young tree or simply as a flexible pole. As you exhale, stop for a moment at the end of the exhalation and just feel the steady centeredness of that column. It remains steady as you inhale and then exhale again, coming back to the stillness between the breaths at the end of each exhale. Now as you inhale, begin a subtle spiral movement with your torso and the inner column that gets larger as you slowly inhale and then gradually gets smaller again as you exhale, until it comes back to stillness and centeredness at the end of the exhale. Once again as you inhale, begin the subtle spiral movement growing larger with the inhalation and then gradually diminishing again with the exhalation. Continue to feel this spiral expanding and contracting with the inhalation and exhalation. When you are ready, add the silent repetition of Om Namah Shivaya as the breath comes in and the spiral expands, and Om Namah Shivaya as the breath goes out and the spiral comes back to stillness. Continue to do this for twenty minutes and then let go of making the movement happen. Just watch how Shakti wants to move or remain still. Enjoy her gifts.

TURIYA: FULLY EXPANDED MEDITATION

The deepest state of meditation, turiya, the transcendent state of the Infinite, is a state unlike the discontinuous states of consciousness that we're familiar with; turiya is continuous. Discontinuous means that if you're in the waking state, you're not in the dream state, if you're in the dream state, you're not in the deep sleep state; they're discontinuous. But when you go into the state of profound meditation, the state of your true nature, it transcends and subsumes these other three states. It's a state that is continuous and, again, with the conditioned mind-brain, when something is continuous, it has the deeply ingrained habit of shutting such things out. When we go past that deeply conditioned mind, we can discover that there's an already present continuous state of meditation available to us that's informed, infused with the irreducible qualities of that Consciousness—the sublime ecstasy, the boundless compassion, the all-embracing love. These aren't produced by the mind or body; these are fundamental to the nature of pure Consciousness.

Because turiya subsumes the other states, you have the capability to be awake meditatively while going about everyday activities. You can be awake meditatively and watch your dreams unfold. You can be awake meditatively and even see your body lying in the depths of deep sleep or physically paralyzed in dream states. I've had students tell me they were terrified by that experience at first because the body was paralyzed; they couldn't move it until they could awaken the ordinary mind out of the dream state to get their body to move. Once they knew that Kundalini had spontaneously given them the experience of being awake and aware while watching the dream state they received the experience as a gift of grace.

Turiya is an already existent state that the practices and awakened Kundalini are bringing you to so that you can eventually be continuously aware of it. It is a state of complete silence and unimaginable stillness within which the whirling energies of the entire universe swirl like a galaxy in a small corner of the Infinitude. But the ego mind fears utter, total stillness. In stillness, in the complete silence of deep meditation, the ego ceases to exist. It fears that and needs to be reassured that it will continue to be summoned into existence, and that it's right action, right service will be appreciated. As long as the physical, subtle, and causal bodies remain, the ego will remain. It can rest assured about this and not fear death. The transcendent, ever-present stillness of boundless, spacious awareness envelops and penetrates the mind-body at all times. Awakened Kundalini immerses us in that awareness over and over and over. We then discover that turiya, the state of Shakti Consciousness, informs and transforms all the other states of consciousness. That state is the foundation of radical freedom.

What is radical freedom? It's going completely beyond the deepest layers of conditioned mind, beyond avidya to the state of the Self, turiya. It's the ability to be informed by our true nature and then have that radiate through our actions, our thoughts, our words, our deeds in whatever state the mind is in. This totally transforms the vehicles of the body and mind so that the contracted emotional states of anger, fear, distress, and feelings of lacking one thing and wanting another, begin to fall away; they are totally incongruent with what your real nature is. The less they are engaged, the more these patterns simply dissolve. You already abide in a fullness and a completeness, a holiness, and wholeness; it's such an extraordinary completeness that once you know it, you see that the other states of the ordinary mind are like a distant phantasm, or a convention one adopts like going to the theatre and suspending ordinary reality in order to enter the drama of the play. From the state of turiya, one sees the play of the mind, the body, and relationships and how they can be informed by the wisdom of the Self, infused with the boundless Love of the Self and express the limitless joy of the Divine embracing life as it is, as its Self.

Until Shakti opened the heart of my heart and tossed me into the ocean of Love, I had no idea what the mystics and yogis were saying when they spoke of the boundless ecstasy and Love of the Self. I dismissed it as hyperbole. I was so wrong, so cut off from the divine reality. Grace has brought me to my knees and stretched me out, face in the ground, sobbing with such an overwhelming sense of Love—being loved, loving, and awed by the majesty of the Loving One who invites us to dissolve in that Love. Nothing but Love, words can't describe it. Words fail to tell how that softens and expands into the awareness of Love throbbing just below the surface of every moment, every creature, everything in this universe.

CHOOSE LOVE

If you take what the Buddha and Christ said,
and all the great yogis, saints, sages,
mystics, and lovers of God,
it can be reduced to two words:
Choose Love.
There is nothing higher than Love,
nothing purer,
nothing more selfless,
nothing more powerful,
and it is present in every moment.

Choose Love.
In all times, in all places -
Choose Love,
for Love has already chosen you.

KALIDAS[2]

MANTRA MEDITATION

As we've discussed, Kundalini takes the vibratory form of mantra. In sadhana the sacred empowered mantras imbued with Kundalini Shakti transform the mind into a vehicle of service and transform consciousness from ordinary states to the sublime state of our infinite being. As Kundalini unfolds, many people have the experience of suddenly hearing inner sounds or seeing inner lights—all are inner vibrations of Shakti. Mantra is a deceptively simple way for the mind to slip into meditation. Mantra gives the mind a handle on a state that transcends it. The mind takes hold of mantra to move beyond itself, beyond its limitations and pain. Kundalini reaches out as mantra and takes hold of the mind to set it free.

I've seen many people with many different backgrounds have spontaneous experiences of hearing inner sounds or having the mantra propel their awareness into unusual states. Often these are people who have had absolutely no experience, no knowledge, and haven't even heard of inner sounds, lights, or visions.

Shortly after the tragedy of 9/11, I was invited to give a program for a group of high school teachers in the area where I lived, just north of New York City. It was to help them with the extreme stress that they had experienced through the school year in trying to help their students deal with the losses they encountered because of the number of deaths. In the program, I taught the use of meditation as a stress management tool. Meditation is taught in many different contexts and is useful in many different areas of life. I taught meditation as a way of entering into profound relaxation and ease, shedding stress and getting beyond the mind that can cause or sustain the stress. I made use of the mantra Om Namah Shivaya. For many people, when they try to just close their eyes and relax, they're confronted by the busy mind and all the things that it does. Taking hold of the mantra is a way of giving the mind a place for attention to settle and allowing it to let go of all the thoughts of the day or whatever else might be going through it. Mantra serves as a kind of vehicle for letting go. I just talked to the high school teachers in that kind of way, and said, "You can focus on the mantra; it'll help ease the mind and calm the mind. We'll chant it for a few minutes, and then we'll sit in silent meditation and during that time, just continue saying the mantra Om Namah Shivaya, Om Namah Shivaya silently over and over in your head and just watch, watch what happens."

They were all totally new to meditation. We did about five minutes of chanting and ten minutes of meditation. As I watched the teachers while they were meditating after we chanted, I noticed one teacher was clearly showing signs that something was going on and towards the end of the meditation, tears were streaming down her face. I rang the gong, and we chanted a couple of rounds of Om Namah Shivaya upon coming out of meditation. Afterward a number of the teachers said, "That felt so nice. I feel so much more relaxed and at ease," but this particular teacher, who looked to be in her fifties, hadn't said anything yet.

Finally at the end she spoke, "I have to say something. You know, I'm a high school teacher. I'm a science teacher. I've taught science for decades now, and I did just what you told me to do; I closed my eyes, I repeated Om Namah Shivaya. I chanted along with you and then kept doing what you said to do after the chanting stopped, just keep silently repeating the mantra. Suddenly I had this experience of a lit-up triangle in the middle of my head, pointing downward, and that triangle seized my awareness, and I went down into my body! I had this view where I could see all the way down into the cells of my body! I'm a science teacher. I could see the cells and their nuclei! I could see the workings of the cells! And I'm going, how could this be? I'm watching everything unfold. (Her voice is getting louder and more excited.) Then, I don't know why, suddenly my awareness in this triangle turned and shot up out of my body, out the top of my head! The next thing I know, I'm streaming through this black void. But then I notice, there are lights flying by. What are those lights? They're stars! I'm out in the middle of the universe; stars are shooting by faster and faster until my vision becomes flooded with light, and that's all there is—light! I disappeared into the light! It was all so beautiful, so moving. The next thing I know I hear the gong! What happened? What am I going to tell my husband? What happened? Something happened, and it moved me to tears, and I was in tears as I came out of this meditation. What happened?"

What happened was she experienced the power of mantra, just sitting with a group of teachers on a sunny afternoon in a nice room in Armonk, New

York. And though she had never studied the esoteric yogic traditions that talk about what's known as the a-ka-tha triangle, that's what she experienced. It's a luminous triangle that exists above your ajna chakra, the third eye, that space between the eyebrows and below your sahasrara (the crown of the head). In there, in the subtle body, is a luminous triangle that is a vehicle for consciousness. It's said that it empowers consciousness to know the universe from the microcosm to the macrocosm. The science teacher had never heard anything like that, but the power of Consciousness encoded in the vibration of mantra gave her that experience. That's Kundalini in the form of mantra, empowering individual consciousness to know the entire grandeur of the universe, from the tiniest workings of a cell to the fields of light and beyond that make up the cosmos. In that instant, the science teacher had the experience of unfolding through the power of Consciousness, the power of mantra, an experience of a rare meditative state that yogis may spend countless years preparing to enter by doing intense practices to refine their consciousness. Taking refuge in empowered mantra—one of the sublime gifts of Kundalini—can give us a taste of magnificent freedom, the freedom of Universal Consciousness, at any moment.

Understanding the power of mantra and the power of words to create reality is also part of what is illumined by Kundalini. She reveals how She creates the reality we experience. Words and how we think shape and create our reality. As I mentioned previously, in the Shaivite tradition, the power of the Shakti to create reality through letters, words, and thoughts is called *matrika shakti,* "little mother power." The little mothers of our thoughts give birth to reality. If I think I'm happy, "I'm happy, I'm happy, I'm happy," it begins to influence my consciousness. If I dwell on, "Life is miserable, I can't stand it," those words shape my reality. Moment by moment we're creating reality by the inner workings of matrika shakti, the power of words, to shape and form our experiences and perceptions that even on a mundane level we need to be attentive to and learn to control.

When we immerse the mind in mantra, we're keeping the mind from going into the old patterns of matrika shakti, the old patterns of thought and habit that create limited realities and the suffering that goes with it. We also can take hold of the patterns of thought to create more expansive realities. When we're saying a mantra like Om Namah Shivaya or Hamsa, it's important to say it with the awareness of "I am Shiva, I am the Infinite, I am the absolute." If you're repeating Om Kali Ma, say it with the awareness of "I am Kali, I am that sublime infinite throb of Consciousness that takes the form of the mantra, that takes the form of the universe, that takes the form of body and mind. The mantra is Kali, the universe is Kali, I am Kali."

We use thoughts and thinking as part of sadhana, cultivating ways of thinking that support our expanding consciousness. In the same way, Buddha talked about the power of mind and the power of thought to create reality. In the Dhammapada, a collection of Buddha's sayings, he says, "Our life is shaped by our mind. We become what we think."[3] Thus, pain and pleasure are as inseparable from our thoughts as heat and light are from fire.

What are the thoughts you are giving your attention to? By giving your attention to them, you're giving them their power to create reality. When there are old thought forms and patterns that we want to pull the energy out of, we need to keep pulling our attention away from them and put our attention and our power into the kinds of thought forms and into the mantra that will transform the reality we're creating. That's how we can transform the mind moment by moment. That's how Shakti empowers us to know radical freedom. Buddha put it succinctly: "as you think so you become." You are responsible for your creation. Kundalini gives you the power and means for re-creating your life.

The simple clear light of awareness, pure unbounded Consciousness, without even a sense of being defining it—this is your nature, this is where your freedom lies. That unbounded awareness is known in silence, in stillness. That's the stillness against which all the movements of the mind are perceived, whether those movements are thoughts or feelings, memories or images, intuitions or realizations—they all rest on that stillness, that expansiveness of pure awareness. We can dial in to that, we can open our consciousness to that awareness, which is the throb of Shakti; that's the throb of Kundalini illuminating all that is. She is that light of awareness that allows us to perceive whatever the thoughts, images, sensations, feelings might be. That Self-luminous, pure awareness is Shakti. She becomes the mantra Om Namah Shivaya that too is a throb, a vibration of the Shakti and carries with it that same power to cut through the mind and bring us to the direct experience of who and what we are. What gifts of revelation She will bestow upon you await your discovery!

Mantra serves as a way to harmonize the mind with Kundalini as the mind becomes absorbed in mantra, bringing the mind into congruence with what Shakti Kundalini is working through. Taking refuge in mantra and becoming absorbed in mantra for meditation are central practices in Kundalini sadhana. In fact, many spiritual traditions look at mantra as the key practice of this age.

In Eastern traditions, the cycle of ages has four components to it, and this last cycle that we're in is called *kali yuga*, meaning "the dark age." But one of the most potent practices for everybody to use during this age is mantra. Mantra is probably the most accessible way of immersing the body and mind in the pure vibrations of the Infinite. In a sense it requires the least effort, the least discipline—all we have to do is silently repeat it, or say it out loud, chant the mantra, or even whisper the mantra, absorbing ourselves in the vibration of pure Consciousness that is the mantra.

You can use a mala, a set of beads, and repeat the mantra as your fingers run across the beads, fall asleep running the mantra through the mind, wake up and have the mind rejoin the stream of inner mantra repetition. People put it on their iPods and make it the soundtrack of their life. Nothing is more uplifting than mantra. The vibratory power of mantra goes where no other practice can—right through the muscles and into the very marrow of our bones, bringing its healing and purifying power to every aspect of the body. In the mind as well, there is no dark corner, no unconscious realm that mantra won't penetrate, illumine, and transform.

Mantra practices are so easy for us to engage in, but the potency of the practice goes far beyond the simplicity of it. Mantra is an actual form of the Infinite, of the Divine. Every time you repeat Om Kali Ma you are invoking the presence of Kundalini Shakti in that moment. By engaging in mantra repetition, absorbing the mind in mantra, it helps to transform the mind and give it a place to rest; it comes to rest in the Divine. Mantra provides an anchor to steady the mind as it goes through whatever the purification process is that Kundalini engenders through her kriyas impacting the mind and body. Once the mind becomes sufficiently clear and subtle, you will actually hear mantras arising within you during meditation. The source of all mantras lies within you. Kundalini is that source, and these infinitely potent vibrations are already resounding within you. Mantra is one of Kundalini's greatest gifts to support one throughout life and even for crossing the border at the time of death. Mantra can go where nothing else can.

Om Namah Shivaya is one of the great mantras, the maha mantras. From the Buddhist tradition, we have another maha mantra: Om Mani Padme Hum. These two mantras are six-syllable mantras. You can use them for going into meditation. When you repeat one of them silently and slowly to yourself in union with the breath, once on the in-breath, once on the out-breath, it does a remarkable thing to your breathing process and actually taps into what scientific research has shown to be a resonant frequency connecting your breathing, your heart rate, the brain, and EEG patterns of the brain. The synchrony brings them into harmony in a very powerful way that has cardiovascular benefits, as well as stabilizing benefits for the mind.

There's biofeedback research showing this slow breathing pattern is useful for working with everything from anxiety disorders to PTSD (post-traumatic stress disorder). These two six-syllable mantras bring the breath right into a pattern of approximately five seconds on the inhalation and five seconds on the exhalation. The ancient yogis discovered this thousands of years ago, and we can make use of that same kind of practice, which will further stabilize the mind and body while it's going through anything that it may encounter on the path of Kundalini sadhana. I use this practice in my clinical work with peak performers, marathon runners, business executives, people with test anxiety, and others, and it works very powerfully to calm and steady the nervous system while promoting a focused, clear mind.

There are other very potent mantras, great mantras, such as Om Kali Ma, a mantra that invokes the great goddess Kali. Kundalini Shakti is one of Kali's forms, and Om Kali Ma invokes that power that is already residing within us. Mantra as a form of Kundalini is part of how Shakti works to transform the mind. The mind is comprised of mantra, but a grosser bound form of it. Absorbing the mind in a mantra with awakened Shakti can give shaktipat and help make that process of descent and ascent more graceful, or as graceful as our own karmas, our own past actions and their consequences, will allow them to be. Take refuge in Om Kali Ma every moment and know Her inexhaustible blessings. She has given me unspeakable gifts through Om Kali Ma.

Taking refuge in mantra moment by moment is a very powerful way of supporting the mind and integrating meditative awareness into waking state consciousness. The goal of meditation is continuous meditative wakefulness, continuous turiya awareness that transcends and subsumes the other states of waking, dream, and deep sleep. Mantra serves as a vehicle for the consciousness to reverberate throughout the mind and through all states of consciousness.

There are many challenges that you'll face on the path of Kundalini, on your soul's journey, and taking refuge in the practices and cultivating a steady mind are imperative. Mantra is one of the greatest practices for stabilizing the mind, centering it, and giving it a life preserver for times of challenge and suffering. When Kundalini is moving through the mind and body, stirring up old samskaras and pushing through blockages, mantra makes the process go more quickly and easily. You can listen to chanting CDs, chant it yourself, repeat it silently, visualize it, paint it, draw it, even write it thousands of times in a notebook to help the mind become absorbed in it.

I led a weekend retreat on mantra with a friend from India who was a swami, and in the retreat she gave people the practice of vowing to write thousands of repetitions of Om Namah Shivaya in a notebook to focus and absorb the mind in the mantra. It opened up meditative states for people as they did it. She then took the notebooks back to India and offered them to Ganga Ma, the holy Ganges River. She said that you will find thousands of notebooks full of mantras that have washed up on the banks of the Ganges from peoples' offerings. You can also write the mantra on sheets of paper and then offer them to a fire. In the Tibetan Buddhist tradition, the prayer wheel has millions of repetitions of Om Mani Padme Hum within it. Practitioners believe that by spinning the prayer wheel, you launch the power of all those mantras into the world for the benefit of all beings. Tibetan prayer flags serve a similar purpose.

The inner, silent repetition of mantra is known as the *inner yagna,* the sacred fire that purifies and sets the mind free of all that encumbers it. This is the power of mantra meditation with an empowered mantra. As we repeat the mantra internally, we become immersed in it, in Om Namah Shivaya or in Om Kali Ma. The blazing power of the mantra, the blazing fire of the mantra, Shakti is what sets our consciousness free from all that binds it. Anything of the mind, anything of the body, and anything of the past can be set free by that inner power, the inner sacred fire of mantra. So allow yourself to become immersed in the inner repetition of Om Namah Shivaya or Om Kali Ma. Meditate on them daily. Dissolve all the illusory boundaries separating you from the mantra and from the Infinite. You are a throb of mantra, a pulsation of the Divine. Know that and live in joy!

Once in meditation Shakti asked me, "How many are prepared to dance with fire? Will you embrace the living flame of divine love? Will you leap with ecstatic abandon into the fire of God's love? Will you allow all but your golden essence to be burned away?" At times this is the path of Kundalini—being in that fire with everything familiar being burned away, knowing that we're going to be reduced to that golden radiant essence. Some months later in meditation as I had become immersed in the mantra repeating itself within my awareness, I found myself standing up and facing an extraordinary tower of flames three or four stories high. I was standing on the edge of an abyss, and the fire filled the abyss and rose up as a towering, crackling, roaring inferno. I could feel the scorching heat upon my skin, it was singeing my eyelashes, and in that flame was this ecstatic laughter, the laughter of a woman coming from the flames! It was Shakti; it was coming from the Devi, this ecstatic laughter of the fire dancing and dancing, but inviting me, saying, "This is it; leap in, leap in!"

I stood there on the edge of that abyss feeling the powerful flames rising with a scorching wind and feeling it calling me to dive in, but I could also feel the searing heat of the fire and my mind recoiling in terror. Suddenly, I leapt into the flames and there was an instant of intense pain, and then there was only Light and Ecstasy, Ecstasy and Light—nothing but that. It was as if in that moment the flames burned away everything but my essential nature of Light and Ecstasy—that's all there was; that's all there is; that is what we are. If we can leap into the Divine with the total abandon She inspires, that's what we will know. That's the promise. That's the power of Shakti; that's what She's inviting us to do. And that's what She's empowering us to do; that's what She gives us the energy to do, to make that leap. She'll show us that there is a fire, but we're going to have to choose to leap. Having taken refuge in Her, taken refuge in mantra, we're going to have the courage, we're going to have the power, we're going to have the strength, and we're going to know ourselves as this Infinite dance of ecstasy, love, and light. In that meditation, as that fire of the divine burned away all sense of self, burned away all sense of separation, there was nothing left. There was no mind.

I have no words to report, no experience to speak of. All I know is that some time later the mind did come back, the ordinary mind, but drenched in stillness. A stillness that also can't be spoken of, that the ordinary mind can't know or describe through words. The mind is movement; it is of the nature of movement. The deep stillness, the deep knowing, is forever beyond the mind. The deep stillness, the deep knowing, humbles the mind. And for all the mind's love of words, of scriptures, of poetry and music, that deep place of knowing is beyond them all. Only Shakti can take you into that. I pray She does that over and over for you. What the mind does know is the sublime delight of being drenched in that state. It is reluctant to return to movement—the stillness is addicting. The mind longs to return there over and over. Eventually one comes to the stillness that is never broken, that surrounds every thought and feeling, that embraces every cell of your body, that is self-luminous, radiant with love. You have the wondrous ability to know that right this instant.

The efforts of the mind can take one all the way up to the rarefied realm of ajna chakra, all the way up to the root of mind. But ultimate knowing is beyond that; there the mind ceases, beyond that only Shakti, only the supreme power of Consciousness goes. And in that transcendent realm, even the forms of mantra dissolve and disappear, there's only a throb of Consciousness; there's only the pure unbounded, self-luminous awareness. There are no scriptures, no words, no thing goes there, yet everything emanates from there—that place, that's your true home. That's your source; that's your essential nature. That's the gift of awakening Kundalini, the direct, pure knowing of That. Tat Twam Asi—Thou Art That.

Kundalini Shakti vibrates the universe into existence through mantra, through the vibration of mantra. On the subtlest levels, that vibration is simply a vibration of Consciousness. As it becomes more gross in form, it takes the form of inner sounds; before they've even reached the level of an audible sound, they're vibrating within. And those vibrations can be heard and experienced in meditation. One of the primal vibrations, primal forms of Kundalini as mantra, is the mantra Om. Om is a mantra that serves as a vehicle for drawing the mind back to the original source and has served as an empowering mantra of other mantras. It's the syllable that gives additional power to a mantra, and you often see Om added to another mantra. For instance, Namah Shivaya is a five-syllable mantra, but Om is added to it, so it's Om Namah Shivaya. You see Om in Buddhist mantras, for instance in Om Mani Padme Hum, or Om Tare Tum Soha. The power of Om, the primal mantra, out of which all other mantras emerge, is then used as a way to add that Shakti to another mantra.

There's an entire Upanishad, the Mandukya Upanishad, dedicated to Om—just that one mantra, because there are so many layers of profound meaning and power in it. The mantra Om encompasses all of creation and the whole of the Sanskrit alphabet. It is the One from which spring the many. Om is comprised of the three sounds A, U, M, and silence, because silence too is part of what the mantra expresses. You can see the symbol for the silence, the point of origin and dissolution represented by the bindu, the dot in the Sanskrit Om symbol. Mantra arises out of silence and dissolves into silence. With that, you get the complete cycle of the emergence of creation through to the dissolution of creation in this one mantra, Om.

The sounds that may seem like syllables when broken out into A-U-M, though they aren't really separate, are representative of the three bodies, the vehicles of consciousness. They represent the physical body, the subtle body, and the causal body. The silence is the supracausal body, the transcendent Self. They also represent the states of consciousness that go with those bodies. The waking state goes with the physical body, the dream state goes with the subtle body, and the deep sleep state, that continuous awareness of nothingness, goes with the causal body. Finally, as well as originally, the transcendent state, the stillness, the silence, is the state of turiya. This is the state of transcendent awareness, of deepest meditation, of pure Consciousness. This one syllable, this one mantra

FIGURE 3 SANSKRIT OM SYMBOL

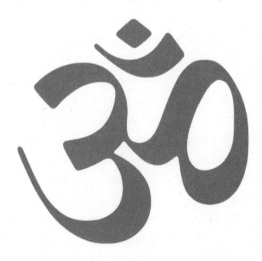

that in our new age culture you see everywhere—in the names of the local yoga center, on bumper stickers—this one sublime mantra encompasses all of creation. This one potent mantra can reveal all that needs to be revealed through its vibration. It is a throb of Consciousness, a throb of Kundalini Shakti vibrating within the sushumna nadi, within you right now. By becoming absorbed in the mantra Om, we can go past the awareness of being identified with the physical body, we can go past the awareness of being identified with the mind and the subtle body, we can even go past the utter blackness of the void of the causal body and enter the Self-luminous awareness, the Infinitude of radiance that is the state of turiya. That is the state of our true, unbounded nature. By following Om, by following this great gift of the Shakti, we can have the direct experience of radical freedom.

In this practice, which is also at the end of the final session of the audio program, we're going to become immersed in that sound of Om, in the inner sound of Om.[4] In this mantra practice, the power of Om dissolves the ordinary mind in its source—Om. This is a practice that was given to me in meditation when Shakti spoke these words that comprise this mantra and this whole meditation. At the end of the practice, we'll be focusing on a chant of the mantra Om, which you can listen to on the program audio or simply repeat in your mind slowly as if chanting it aloud, repeat it over and over again. During that time you can just allow your awareness to become absorbed in the inner sound of Om and watch what unfolds. It may even be that you discover that your awareness goes beyond that sound, goes beyond anything that is of the ordinary mind—and that's the grace of Shakti, the grace of Kundalini, taking your awareness wherever it may need to go. Just allow that to happen and become absorbed in Om.

OM MEDITATION

To begin, allow yourself to adjust and take your best meditation posture, whether it's seated on the floor or a supported upright posture in a chair, whatever allows you to be most comfortable while being alert, aware, and awake. Choose a posture that supports consciousness and awareness. Allow your attention to come to your breath; the breath is one of the first ways that we can engage the process of calming the mind, allowing it to quiet, becoming more still and at ease. With every breath allowing the mind to let go and let go, following the wisdom of the body, just as with every exhalation, the body expels what it most needs to be rid of. So too the mind following the breath can expel and let go of thoughts and feelings, memories, anything that it needs to be free of at this time, in this place. As the mind becomes quieter and more refined, as awareness becomes more subtle, we're able to perceive things that before we may have missed. Just as when you're outside in the bright sun and you walk into a dimly lit room, you can't see a thing. But then, as your eyes adjust, you find you can see quite clearly. In the same way, we detach the mind from all the things of the ordinary world, allow it to rest on the breath, and allow it to simply be present and feel the spaciousness of awareness. It doesn't matter what might be moving through that spaciousness of awareness, whether there are external sounds, whether it's internal movements of the mind; awareness just watches, detached and at ease. The body is invited to let go and let go, even as the mind continues to let go. Beneath all the noise of the mind, underlying all awareness, there's a gentle throb, like a swell in the ocean, a throb of the mantra Om. Om is already vibrating throughout your subtle body and your body.

Shakti said, "When you unfurl a sail to catch the wind, the sail is visible, the wind is not. You use the visible to catch the invisible. You use the perceptible to approach the imperceptible." At first you may sound aloud the word Om over and over again: Om, Om, Om. And in time you will stop sounding Om aloud; continue repeating it silently within your mind. Focus your entire attention on that inner resonance, that inner vibration of Om. There's no audible sound, yet your consciousness reverberates with that un-struck sound of Om, Om, Om. In time subtler vibrations of consciousness may replace the sound vibrations; the subtle vibrations of consciousness dissolve the mind, dissolve even the inner sound of Om. And the vibrations of consciousness can become finer and finer, more and more subtle, until they become light, pure shimmering light, the pure light of Consciousness, the light of the Divine. And there you are in the presence of the Light. Just be still, no effort is needed. Your consciousness is being drawn nearer and nearer to the Divine. Here you wait—in the glory and the light of God, waiting for the Divine to pull your consciousness into union with the Infinite. And the Divine finally draws you in, and with that act of grace, you move beyond all words and descriptions, beyond perceiver and perceived, beyond experience and experiencer, beyond even love and ecstasy. This is your true home, your true refuge. Step into the light, step into the light as often as you can. Allow the Lord to draw you near and scoop you up in his arms. Your soul cries out for the loving embrace of the divine. Don't deny yourself that love any longer. Dissolve into that loving embrace. Dissolve into that love and light. Om arises out of that stillness and dissolves into that stillness. Om, the sublime vibration, your own infinite awareness, leads the mind back, back into the realm of form, but infused with the Light of Consciousness, infused with the vibration of Om. As you listen to that sound of Om in the chant, allow that sound to vibrate throughout the body, throughout the mind, opening awareness to that vibration of Om that already lies within. Dissolve the mind in that sound of Om.

Living radically free is living our innate, unimpeded power to give boundless love, boundless compassion, patience, wisdom, and strength to all in need, to effortlessly radiate these qualities to all around you.

May all our practices truly benefit everyone, and may all beings now know complete freedom from suffering.

12

The Role of the Teacher/Guru in Kundalini Sadhana

Several years ago Shakti began appearing to me in meditations as Tara, one of the divine feminine forms in Tibetan Buddhism. She told me to receive initiation into the Tara tradition, though at that time I knew very little about Tara, and I certainly didn't know anyone in that tradition. My Devi was very insistent and said I should learn about Tara and specifically Red Tara and Black Tara. For many years Shakti had been teaching me from within as Kali and had taught me about other forms of the dark Goddess, including Inanna and the Black Madonna. It made sense that She would extend this into Tara's realm. In this inner dialogue with Kali Shakti, I said I would need Her to provide a way for me to receive these initiations and teachings. Since it was Her will that this happen, I completely trusted that somehow it would.

Several months later a woman contacted me about Kundalini experiences she had been having and wanted to consult with me about them. We spoke on the phone a couple of times, and then she flew out to New York to meet with me. As her story unfolded, it turned out that she had been having a number of different experiences, but one included visions of me, though we had never met. She searched the Internet and found a picture of me, and it matched the picture she had seen in a vision that connected me with her teacher. Her teacher is the great

Buddhist master, His Eminence Tsewang Sitar Rinpoche, the head of the ancient Sangye Teng Monastery in Bhutan. He was visiting a Buddhist community in her city and building a stupa there. Rinpoche is a master in the Tara tradition.

I shared my experience of the Devi telling me to receive initiation into the Tara tradition. She told me about Tsewang Sitar Rinpoche, and I flew out to meet him. He graciously began giving me Tara empowerments and teachings, though there was only his other student and I there. It didn't matter. He knew this was Tara's will. To me, he is a living Buddha. He is as humble as water, as grand as the Himalayas, as powerful as lightning, and as kindly as an old grand-mother. The Devi brought me to him so he could impart those extraordinary Tara teachings to me.

A couple of years later when His Holiness the Dalai Lama had brought H. E. Tsewang Sitar Rinpoche to Miami to give him and his monks empowerments and teachings, Rinpoche generously agreed to come up to New York to give a small group of us empowerments and teachings. He brought the same enthu-siasm, graciousness, humility, and brilliance to us as he did to teaching H. H. the Dalai Lama, his monks, and the throngs of people in Miami. He lives the dharma, and he lives to pass on the dharma. He is a treasure.

There is an old saying, "Thank God for the Guru, for it is the Guru that brings us to God." The One manifests forms within us and outside of us to lead us on our path.

THE GURU / SPIRITUAL MASTER / LAMA

There's so much written on the critical role of the teacher/guru/lama/spiritual director that one could study the texts for many years. If you are already pur-suing a particular tradition, you've probably encountered teachings on this subject. If you are new to yoga and meditative practices, this subject area will become more important as your concentrated efforts deepen. Studying teach-ings on the role of the guru or lama or master is helpful for developing one's discrimination and expectations.

Reading about the lives of great masters and their relationships to their teachers is also invaluable for developing one's discrimination in this area of sad-hana. There are dynamics and teachings that are conveyed in the guru-disciple relationship that occur in no other relationship, and these can be discerned by studying these works. There are also many different styles in which great masters have taught and directed their students. No one teacher and no one tradition embodies all the possibilities. Reading about the lives of Marpa and Milarepa, Tilopa and Naropa, Paramahansa Yogananda, Swami Muktananda, Kabir, Saint Teresa of Avila, Saint John of the Cross, Rumi, Mirabai, Ramakrishna, and many other great mystics will expand and enrich your vision of teacher-student relationship. These are inspired relationships of profound love, commitment, and grace.

The ancient Shiva Sutras offer what may be the most succinct summary statement on the guru: "the guru is the means."[1] The teacher/guru is the means for learning practices, wisdom, and compassion and for seeing freedom, love, and mindfulness embodied and modeled by a living person. Most rarely and importantly the guru is the means for imparting power, Shakti, through mantras, practices, and the loving presence of the master, who directly awakens you to the highest. A true master is one who has been molded by the Divine in the crucible of intense practices and selfless service to form the instrument of grace that the Divine uses to confer blessings and lead seekers back to the source. For these reasons a wise and selfless teacher at some point is essential for progressing on the path.

The Sage Patanjali recommends that the student practice fixing his or her mind on one who has risen above attachment and passion, and in this way the student will imbibe the sublime qualities of the guru as the grace-bestowing power of the Infinite.[2] By doing this dharana, this focusing practice on one who embodies the highest, the mind becomes attuned to those qualities and to the teacher's consciousness. People do this unconsciously with rock stars, athletes, actors, and actresses. Yoga elevates this human propensity to a conscious practice done in the service of transformation and self-realization.

Despite seekers' wishes to be magically and instantly set free, Buddha made it clear that a master can't just give that state of freedom to another. But the master teacher can empower, instruct, guide, and inspire the seeker on the path. You'll discover there are teachers who have only a little to impart and others with whom you could spend lifetimes and not absorb all they have to give.

PROJECTION AND IDENTIFICATION

One of the most important functions of the living master is that they carry the projection of our own highest nature—Self, Buddha, Shakti, Kali—whatever form we love to imagine that to be. The wise master is one who can carry that projection and turn it back to the seeker. This is part of the tantric path. On the tantric path, the deity, guru, or other form is first invoked and related to as separate and different from oneself. Then through practices, visualization, meditation, and identification, one realizes that there is no outer, separate deity, it is all within you as you.

The archetype of the Source, the transcendent One, is singular, an all-encompassing unity. The state of that one is Unity Consciousness. There's just the One who takes on limitations and avidya, ignorance of its own true nature, as well as taking on a limited form for awakening that part from ignorance by transmitting true knowledge and freedom from suffering. The One takes the form of the seeker, searching on their quest, and discovers the One embodied in a teacher. In time, the seeker awakens to the full truth—they are the One and always have been. They are the seeker and the sought, the forgetting and the remembering, and the unspeakable Love, the ground on which the entire creation unfolds. The guru is God serving God through God's love. That is the *ideal*. That's the archetypal form of the relationship. That's the huge power underlying what gets projected to some degree or another on the teacher/lama/guru/priest. It is best to be awake and aware of this dynamic. It informs the ideal and dharma of the roles of both the guru and the disciple/student. However, one also needs to be mindful of the ego posturing at possessing the real knowledge, the fully and directly known wisdom and freedom that comes from genuinely having moved from a place of ignorance and bondage to a place of freedom. The ego mind so likes to pretend and deludes itself in the process!

The ego mind needs to learn how to relate to the Divine. It does this through the guru/master to whom one vows obedience and surrender in the archetypal form of this relationship. The ego mind finds it very difficult to learn how to relate to the Divine within through an abstraction, an idea. It learns through the relationship with the master. (In general the mind learns from the concrete to the abstract.) God, guru, and Self are one. This is why obedience and surrender are demanded. The sadhana of guru yoga or the guru-disciple relationship is ideally meant to cultivate that loving surrender, impeccable obedience, and intuitive readiness to follow the will of the Divine, to follow Shakti Kundalini, in every moment. That's the true dharma of this relationship.

However, there are few masters and few disciples able to be unwavering in their adherence to that dharma. In this age that we live in, dharma is at its lowest ebb everywhere. The psyche projects the Self onto whatever convenient projection screen is around in its attempt to relate to and unite with the Self. That projection screen could be a hatha yoga teacher, a meditation teacher, a therapist, a priest, rabbi, and so forth. Most of these people don't get trained in how to deal with such projections or transference and counter-transference as we call it in the psychological professions. Not that training is sufficient to prevent unconscious acting out! The lack of awareness of the dynamic of projection sets up both the teacher and the student to fall into the unconscious and act out the folly of ignorance creating more suffering, more karma, more rounds of birth and death.

These are very seductive and powerful projections. Teachers who aren't selfless, free of all cravings and desires, and established in the highest, unconsciously or consciously want to be adored as embodiments of wisdom and divinity. Students unconsciously or consciously want someone to carry that projection, and then the student wants to receive loving attention from them, *as if* the student were receiving it from the Divine, Buddha, or God. Sadhana demands that we be awake to this. It is another dynamic of the conditioned mind that binds people for lifetimes. That doesn't mean automatically demeaning the guru-disciple relationship or denigrating masters who respectfully carry such projections in a skillful way and know that everyone is Divine. It means developing discrimination through study, contemplation, self-study, meditation, and seva. Shankaracharya said that one develops discrimination by serving those who have realized the truth.

GURU PRINCIPLE: THE GRACE BESTOWING
POWER OF THE INFINITE

Kshemaraja in his commentary on the Shiva Sutras, says the guru is the grace-bestowing power of God,[3] meaning the true guru is a divine power, not the person it flows through. The guru is Kundalini Shakti. Many times I heard Swami Muktananda speak about the true nature of the guru or the guru principle being the divine power of grace, Kundalini Shakti, flowing through an individual. Shakti is inseparable from the Self; it is the Universal Power of Consciousness. Thus, on the highest level of understanding, it is not the individual who is referred to as the guru, but the universal power, Shakti manifesting through an individual. The essential nature of the highest guru is transpersonal, not individual. In this way the true guru/master is the inner guru, the archetypal power of the Self-revelation; in yogic terms it is Kundalini.

The word guru points to the idea that a teacher is one who leads a seeker from the darkness of ignorance to the light of wisdom. The first syllable, *gu,* means "darkness"; the second syllable, *ru,* means "light." Just as there are different forms of darkness and ignorance and different levels of light and wisdom, so too there are different types and levels of gurus and teachers. It's said that one's parents are one's first gurus. You would go to a *tabla* (percussion instrument) guru to learn to play the tablas, but for Kundalini, you would seek the assistance of one graced by Kundalini to impart Her wisdom.

The ability to awaken Kundalini can be seen in accomplished masters of many traditions. There have been great Christian saints whose touch or words inflamed the souls of those who followed them. Similarly there have been rabbis, Sufi masters, yogis, and Buddhist masters awakening people and giving empowerments, dharma transmissions, and initiations based on conveying the power of wisdom and grace.

Though the Guru principle is archetypal, transpersonal, the power of the Divine, that doesn't mean the individual who is embodying that principle or carrying the projection of it is infallible or perfect. We have to use our discrimination when looking at the human form of the guru. The savvy seeker is wary of the shadow sides of gurus, which are often hidden or obscured by the brilliance of the light of ancient truths they clothe themselves in. We have to look past the public persona of the guru to see what they truly embody. There's a dharma to being a student as well as a dharma to being a teacher. Both need to be observed.

Imagine that you've wandered across a seemingly endless desert, and you are literally dying of thirst when you come upon a humble abode, inside of which there is a simple faucet. You turn on the faucet, and life-saving water flows out. You can't believe your good fortune! You drink your fill and rest there for a while, gathering strength for the remainder of your journey. You might have tremendous gratitude for the one who built the shelter and for the well and faucet for making the life-saving water available to you, but as you leave, taking a jug with you, you don't stop and build a shrine to the faucet. You don't bring your journey to an end there in order to spend the rest of your life worshipping the faucet, though you may well tell everyone who's thirsty where they can be refreshed. On your spiritual journey across the arid desert of avidya, when you encounter the guru, the master, through whom the life-saving wisdom of dharma, through whom Kundalini Shakti flows, know that they are like that faucet, and Shakti, in one form or another, is the water flowing through them. Appreciate them for having become the empty, holy conduit for grace and know that it is the water of grace that saved you and refreshed you, empowering you to finish your journey. Some faucets are cleaner and purer than others and don't impart any aftertaste to the sweet waters of grace pouring through them. Use your discrimination to discern this. At the end of your journey, perhaps Shakti will turn you into a humble faucet, forever resting in the open position.

THE INNER GURU

On the highest level, the guru/teacher is Kundalini Shakti, which is working from within on all levels to bring about the radical freedom that is your birth-right, and working from the outside, through individuals serving as teachers/ guides, sometimes even unknowingly or through situations that occur on your soul's journey, which demand mastery of skills, knowledge, courage, and selflessness. For Shakti, there is no inside-outside duality—all lies within Her, within the body of the Divine. Thus, in Kundalini sadhana, we have to develop the discrimination to see the workings of the grace-bestowing power of the Divine, Kundalini Shakti, the primal guru present at all times, in all places. She is *sat;* She is eternally true.

In this book, I've focused on the inner guru, the workings of Kundalini, and how to understand and follow Her mysterious ways. Because it is so dif-ficult to differentiate between the promptings of Kundalini and the ego mind on many levels, a trusted teacher and guide is necessary in Kundalini sadhana to prevent one from getting lost in the maze of mind-born interpretations of Shakti's directions.

DISCRIMINATION: IMPORTANT FACTORS
FOR CHOOSING A TEACHER

In Kundalini sadhana, as in all sadhanas, at some point it becomes essential to have a teacher or a guide, somebody who is deeply practiced, thoroughly trained, selfless, and compassionate. The relationship that develops with a genuine teacher differs from all other relationships we'll ever have. The dharma of a teacher is unique, as well as the dharma of a genuine student or disciple.

How a teacher becomes a teacher is important. In an ancient traditional context, one went to the teacher solely to become free. You would go to the teacher, the master yogi, Rinpoche, or lama simply to become free. Not to get a certificate, not as a career choice, not to be made into a teacher or a guru—you go to become free. To *become* anything else is to be less than free; it just keeps the ego mind's game of becoming this and identifying with that going on and on. One has to shed all becoming. Eventually, once the students are free, the master may instruct some to become teachers, and some might still be out in the field doing the seva of picking up cow dung. But because they're free, they can do whatever seva they are given with the full delight that's within them wherever they are. One seva isn't better than another. Though being free empowers them to serve others in a unique way as a true teacher and to pass on that freedom is part of their seva, their surrender to dharma. They will transmit teachings no matter where they are or what they do. There are *avadhuts,* "enlightened beings" in India, whose life is the teaching, even if it comes through them while they live naked atop a garbage heap as Zipruanna Baba (a contemporary of Muktananda) did.

Sage Patanjali instructed seekers to take refuge in a teacher who is selfless, who has risen above attachments and cravings. Such a one needs nothing from you. They can't be manipulated by your ego mind or unconsciously collude with the ego by feeding it in order to hold onto you. I met a swami from India who was telling me how her guru had instructed her in becoming a guru, and one of the things he taught her was how to hook students and disciples so they would support her. It was shocking and very revealing about the shadow sides of some traditions.

These days developing the stature of gurus, lamas, teachers, and the like has been greatly influenced by market forces and competition for attention and money. That is the realm of the ego mind. Is it any wonder then that so many teachers, once elevated by such market forces and ego drives, are subsequently found to require further spiritual development? People want yoga teacher certificates as a career choice. Then, some scramble to develop a brand and their own form of yoga that they can market along with a stylish line of yoga clothes.

What does this have to do with becoming free and helping others to become free? It's fine as exercise and wellness routines, but true yoga is solely about becoming free.

Remember that as student or a seeker, you have to develop the discrimination to discern what's useful that you can learn from a teacher and what's not. What does this particular teacher have to give and what needs to be left behind or doesn't go far enough? Very often people going through Kundalini processes are in a vulnerable state. They may be in a state of panic, they may be in a state of pain, they may be in a state of confusion, and they're desperately seeking somebody to help them. This can set a person up to either consciously or unconsciously be taken advantage of by others. It's very important to have a kind of vigilance and mindfulness about the nature of a teacher and what one is seeking from the teacher. Bring your discrimination to evaluating a teacher. You are entrusting them with a critical role in your journey that will have an impact on this life and future lives. Consider this carefully. How well trained are they? How experienced are they? What is this teacher really about? What are they demanding? A genuine teacher teaches in a way that engenders respect, even if they can be blunt or pointed at times; it is only in service of the student progressing or breaking through something. Good teachers are respected for the love, wisdom, and guidance they give, the patience and compassion that they live. They don't get respect because of a power trip, because they demand blind loyalty, because they want to dominate others or engender fear. If a teacher is exhibiting any of those kinds of patterns, then you know that their shadow side has not been cleared and you're in danger. Use your discrimination; leave if necessary.

There are teachers offering powerful yogic or spiritual practices unaware that those practices may lead to Kundalini awakening and are caught off-guard when one of their students has a sudden awakening. I have heard from both teachers and students who have had this experience. In 1972, I took a type of Kundalini yoga course for months that involved a great deal of vigorous asanas and pranayama along with chanting and other practices. I began having very unusual meditative experiences that visibly scared the yoga teacher when I told him about them. He had no idea what they meant or how they were related to the practices. He was ignorant, and I was ignorant. I stopped doing the practices, and the challenging events ceased. They marked some stirrings of prana and quickly passed.

It's important for seekers to know they're empowered to use their discrimination to see clearly and to know for themselves what is going to be of genuine support and to know when the situation is toxic and they need to leave it. Too often, the ego mind is seeking magical ways to get out of its pain. It brings that desire to teachers. It's looking for somebody who is going to say, "Oh, I can just do this, that, or the other thing, and your practices will be effortless," and we need to be wary of that. Even Buddha, after becoming enlightened under the Bodhi tree, got up and stood back from where he had sat, reflecting on his experience. His first impulse was to walk away, feeling a tragic sense that he could never give that experience away, could never simply pass it on to others. All the gods and goddesses came to him and begged him to in some way try to teach it. Buddha reflected for a while and thought something like, "Well, it's true. I can't just pass this experience on, but I can teach a method. I can teach a way by which people can come to realize this for themselves, to become free of suffering themselves."

We have to walk our own path. We have to walk through the experiences that the unfolding of our karma demands. A good teacher can help guide your steps, can help support, encourage, and test you. They can give practices that sustain progress and steady the mind. But they can't magically make all challenges disappear. And this is something that's important for seekers to remember, especially those going through difficult Kundalini processes. The ordinary mind wants to get out of pain as quickly as possible. In fact, everybody wants to get out of pain—that's what motivates us to get free of suffering. But we have to walk our path and do our practices, informed by what awakened Kundalini can give as well as by genuine teachers. Having been through the process themselves, true teachers can share insights that will support, encourage, and empower us to continue on our way.

Kundalini awakening accelerates and brings to fruition yoga and meditation practices. From a yogic perspective, that means the difference between living countless lifetimes of evolution or only a few. That's a huge change in pace! But to the ego mind that would like freedom and enlightenment in a weekend retreat or maybe in a few years if one is really patient, the notion of lifetimes is too much. It makes most people run to find someone who will tell them that they can have it all now. That is possible if you've done the lifetimes of sadhana to be at the point where you fall into radical freedom like perfectly ripe fruit dropping off a tree with the barest touch. But most people need more time to bask in the radiance of the Self, of Buddha mind, to finish ripening. The practices, the teachings, the teacher, and fellow seekers keep one in the Light.

THE TEACHER'S ROLE BEFORE AND AFTER AWAKENING

The role of the teacher before Kundalini awakening differs from their role afterward. Prior to the awakening of Kundalini, the teacher offers instruction on the path that they have traveled to gain direct knowledge themselves. They may teach practices for awakening Kundalini (pranayama, mantra, Classical yoga, etc.), and if they are one of the rare teachers who can truly pass on Kundalini empowerment, serving as a conduit for shaktipat, then the student is especially fortunate. After Kundalini awakening, a skilled teacher works to guide and safeguard a seeker on the path. In Kundalini sadhana, you might have the one teacher from whom you received shaktipat or whose teachings and practices you follow closely, while at the same time there may be additional teachers who impart other valuable practices or empowerments. You might learn hatha yoga from one teacher, Vedanta from another, and mindfulness from yet another, all while being guided by your root guru or main teacher.

Once Kundalini awakens, a whole new play between the inner teacher and the outer teacher unfolds. This play can only fully unfold with a truly wise and surrendered master teacher. What occurs then is so sublime it can barely be spoken of. It is the play of Shiva and Shakti, Lover and Beloved, reveling in unity, delighting in creation, enveloping all in loving compassion and incomparable grace. In this age where *adharma* ("not in accord with the law," the opposite of dharma) is so prevalent and afflicted teachers abuse and mislead students, the exquisitely grace-filled relationship with a true dharmic teacher is harder to find. More and more discrimination is demanded of seekers. Oh, but how the heart blossoms in the presence of such a selfless compassionate one! It's good to be wary, but please don't become cynical and close-hearted. Keep your eyes open. The grace-bestower walks this earth in many forms and may be closer than you realize.

I am so indebted to the extraordinary masters I've had the great good fortune to learn from and receive empowerments from. Even with all future lives dedicated to serving and passing on their gifts, there is no way to repay them or adequately express the overwhelming gratitude that comes with their gifts.

Even the capacity to feel such humbling gratitude is a gift of grace. There's nothing for the ego mind to appropriate, to take credit for. This gratitude arises from the pure Love radiating from Light of Wisdom within the heart, lit by the Devi through Her forms of inner and outer guru. Jai Ma!

13

Upayas

The Means to Freedom

All of the foundational practices that I've written about are aimed at bringing the mind and our actions into congruence, into harmony with where Shakti is leading us. Meditation, Witness Consciousness, self-inquiry, Classical yoga, and similar practices all help clear the mind and the body so that we can live ever more present within that awareness of our Infinite nature and the Divine nature of everyone and everything. The Shiva Sutras give a profound yet practical way of looking at the different practices that we engage in to support that expanding awareness of Shakti Consciousness.

The Shiva Sutras categorize the entire range of practices into three upayas, or "means." The practices are the means that we engage in to change our awareness and consciousness in the moment. The upayas classify the practices and make it clear how they match where we are in the moment. In the Shiva Sutras, the upayas are delineated starting with the most subtle ones appropriate for near Unity Consciousness states and working their way to the upaya dealing with the other end of the spectrum, the state of duality and separation. We'll start by looking at that upaya and work toward the subtler and subtlest upayas.

BEDA UPAYA

The first upaya we'll discuss is *beda upaya,* also known as *anavopaya.* Beda upaya practices are used when we're in a state of duality or difference. We experience ourselves as different and separate from the Divine, the Self. *Beda* means "difference." We may feel no real consciousness of being directly connected to the Divine, and the practices from beda upaya are ways of bringing our mind and our attention closer to the Divine, but they start with that sense of separation. For instance, if we're going about our day (and it could be right from when we wake up in the morning) and we're thinking, "Oh, I've got to go do this and that," then it's likely we're not even thinking about our sadhana or our connection to the Divine in the moment nor experiencing unity with the Divine in any way. There are practices that take us from the experience of being caught in forgetfulness or caught in separation from our Self and bring consciousness back to the goal of sadhana, the direct experience of the Divine moment by moment. These practices can be everything from devotional practices, lighting a candle and looking at an image of the Divine, chanting, or doing mantras, but we may be engaging in the practices from that state of feeling separate.

As you become immersed in a beda upaya practice, it starts to refine your attention. It starts to refine the mind and draw it closer to that experience of, "Oh, that divinity really is inside of me. I feel the stirrings of that. I feel the connectedness to that." In this way, the beda upaya practices start with that sense of difference and aim at helping to dissolve it so we can come closer to the Divine. Practices like offering whatever we're doing as an offering of seva, of selfless service to the Divine, is a beda upaya practice. It's a beautiful practice, and it helps to transform the ego mind that comes out of a sense of separation, but now through the practice, it relates to the Divine and connects with the Infinite through love and dedication.

Beda upaya practices include many of the things that we think of as yoga practices, for instance the hatha yoga asanas and breathing exercises of pranayama. These are all aimed at helping to transform the mind and the body to be vehicles that hold that awareness. They start off with the feeling of separation, which dissolves over time into Unity Consciousness. Other practices include prostrations. In the Tibetan Buddhist tradition, one can make vows of doing prostrations by the hundreds of thousands and even millions of times.

This is a beda upaya practice that transforms the mind and body into a humble, devoted servant, a surrendered servant, by entering into this physical posture of surrender and adoration. Even practices like contemplation and study, studying the scriptures, reading the words of the Buddha, and studying Patanjali's Yoga Sutras are beda upaya practices aimed at transforming the mind through wisdom and helping it become more attuned and connected to the Divine.

The wisdom practices and ethical practices of the Noble Eightfold Path are beda upaya practices. All these different practices start with that sense of separation and aim at moving toward union. We can do this in our relationships, even when we're looking at our spouse or our loved ones and they seem so separate. We can literally do a dharana, a focusing practice of imagining them as the embodiment of the Divine and seeing them with all the love and devotion that we might bring to an image of the Buddha, Christ, or an image of a god or goddess. By incorporating an image of the Divine into our vision of a loved one near us, we are serving them as we would the Divine. That's a beda upaya practice.

Sometimes beda upaya techniques have to do with physically having things in our environment that we encounter throughout the day that help to remind us of our connection, of the Divine present at all times. A picture on a wall, a saying on our computer screen, a statue on our dashboard—these are beda upaya techniques. They're perfectly valid. They help the mind physically encounter a reminder so it can say to itself, "Oh yeah, that's right, that's here. I can come back to that. I like having a laughing Buddha greeting me as I walk in the door!" Whatever your choice of what that reminder looks like, you are using a beda upaya technique. Dualistic traditions limit themselves to beda upaya practices of prayer, viewing icons, contemplations, service to others, rosaries, pilgrimages, and so forth.

As that state of difference, of separation, begins to dissolve, we might find ourselves in meditation, having perhaps started with a beda upaya practice of chanting out loud, or saying a mantra in our mind, but with a sense that there's a difference between the mantra, the source of the mantra, and the Divine. These three appear to be separate. As they start to merge, as they start to melt together, there comes a point where we can begin to use our mind and shaktopaya, the next upaya, which has to do with how we use our mind to dissolve boundaries, differences, and the illusion of separation.

SHAKTOPAYA

Shaktopaya is also known as *beda-abeda upaya,* "difference and non-difference means." It refers to the state of consciousness in which difference and separation have diminished, and non-difference and union are beginning to emerge. For instance, if we're doing a mantra practice, and we've gotten past the beda upaya level separation and the boundaries that seem to separate the mantra, and the source of the mantra and our being all begin to dissolve, then we're in the space of consciousness where shaktopaya techniques are used. The mantra as a separate sound form isn't even there. We can begin to see that as the boundaries dissolve, we settle into the actual direct experience of union, of merger with the mantra. You can begin to feel "I am the mantra; I am this throb of Consciousness, of Shakti that is mantra." Now, we're entering the state where we can draw on the mind as consciousness; the forms of body and ordinary mind are dissolving into consciousness. There's only an indescribably thin veil separating us from entry into a deeper, fuller mystical state of union. We're actually using consciousness, bare awareness devoid of an "I" or ego sense, to focus on the unspeakable Presence. Then, as that experience unfolds, we merge. The body may be sitting or even moving (it's not just during sitting meditation that this happens), but for most people, it's during sitting meditations that they will begin to experience this stage of merger and union. Later on, it is going to blossom and become something that you experience even in the midst of activity.

Sitting meditation practices are really aimed at helping us to dial into the direct experience of this Unity Consciousness, but not that it's only available when we're sitting with our eyes closed or staring at the ground. Living samadhi is the state that Shakti Kundalini is unfolding. This living samadhi is referred to in the Shiva Sutras as *lokananda samadhi sukham*—the bliss of the world is the bliss of samadhi.[1] It's a living state of ecstasy that encompasses all of life, all the world. But we practice entering that state in the quieter practice of sitting meditation. In the Buddhist tradition, we say nirvana is samsara, and samsara is nirvana. This conveys the same point that the highest attainment dissolves the boundary between what appears to be separate, even opposed states.

Meditation as a process cultivates an expansiveness that allows one to genuinely transcend and subsume that boundary. When you plant a tree and cultivate it in a greenhouse, it grows and gains strength in a protected environment.

You'll finally have to harden it off to plant it outside where it will thrive in the elements and grow into its fullness as a tree. Meditation practice is like that protected process. Because the mind is so used to going after all the distractions, it needs the reduced sounds, darkened room, and stillness that we create in meditation. But that's not the end state. Meditation as a state isn't fragile. It can't be broken. It's the mind's steadiness that is fragile to begin with. Its focus and stillness is easily broken at the beginning of one's practice.

In shaktopaya, as we become familiar with drawing close to that experience of merger and union and as there's a letting go of the thoughts, concepts, and wisps of the ego mind (it's the ego mind that holds onto a limited state of I-ness, a limited identity that goes with each thought or perception), we then get to a place of just using the mind to let go of all that. Then there's dissolution into that Light of Consciousness. There's a greater light than the mind; there's the Light of Consciousness itself that illumines all that is and invites merger with your Self.

SHAMBHAVOPAYA

You can draw so close to complete union that you're then in a state where *shambhavopaya* is used (though *used* is too gross a term since there is no real form of ego mind or self present to do or use anything). *Shambho* is Shiva, the Self, the bestower of unshakeable peace. Shambhavopaya is almost no means at all; because it is so subtle and so refined, there's nothing as gross as an action of the mind or personal will. There's nothing as coarse as a thought or an imagining; shambhavopaya is the barest movement of intention, even subtler than that, so subtle that words can't describe it. It may be thought of as pure grace that pulls consciousness into Consciousness, like a magnetic force that is invisible, indescribable, but potent. Its irresistible power reveals that you are already enveloped; you are already united; there never was a time when you weren't. Bliss reigns supreme! It is pure union, but so far beyond words the mind weeps at its failure to convey anything about this state. In this sublime state, there's no longer thought; there's no longer the movement of thought. If even a hint of thought arises, then you re-engage shaktopaya. If the movement from a samskara, an old pattern of mind, brings you back into the argument that you had yesterday or to what happened on the way to work, then you're back in a state of total separation, and you use a beda upaya practice once again.

The different upayas make it clear that the efficacy of a practice is related to the state we're in. If we're in a state of separation, feeling really different from every-thing and separate from the Divine, not even remembering that it's there, and we use a shambhavopaya approach, it's completely inappropriate because we're not in that state. Shaktopaya techniques may not work either because we're not in proximity to the Divine where just shifting our awareness to dissolve the veil-like boundaries within the mind is going to draw us closer. A beda upaya practice may be called for.

Understanding the upayas also makes it clear that until one is a very accom-plished practitioner, most practices that one engages are beda upaya practices. If all we had to rely on was self-effort, then beda upaya practices might be all we did for many, many lifetimes. Fortunately, awakened Kundalini can spontane-ously, in a moment, temporarily erase all sense of ego self and limited identity and drown one in the ecstatic, all-encompassing state of the Self, of Shiva/Shakti, turiya—words desperately trying to point infinitely beyond themselves. At first She gives you a visitor's visa to let you into transcendent states. When you've become completely pure, worthy of taking up residence there, she'll reveal the truth that no words can speak. Take refuge in Shakti Kundalini, and know this directly for yourself. As your mind becomes more refined and skilled at follow-ing Shakti's guidance, She will reveal more and more to you. Kundalini Shakti is the power of revelation and transformation. Follow her ways and receive all the gifts She wants to bestow upon you.

KUNDALINI SADHANA: ALL-INCLUSIVE GUIDELINES

We've looked at the nature of Kundalini as pure Consciousness and how the eight limbs of Classical yoga as well as the central practices of empowered man-tra, Witness Consciousness, and mindfulness are critical to Kundalini sadhana. We've also discussed the importance of finding and working with a skilled teacher who can impart specific practices, wisdom teachings, and guidance needed for navigating your way along your soul's journey and the magnificent quest you are on.

Kundalini sadhana relies on the grace and direction of Kundalini. It is a fluid and dynamic process that incorporates the overlapping, mutually sup-portive and integrative practices we've been discussing. Prior to Kundalini awakening, you might engage practices from a tradition that safely awakens

Kundalini. You can use mantra, chanting, meditation, or gentle breath work to attune yourself to Shakti. Doing daily practices makes the instrument of the mind more and more subtle, more and more refined, able to hear Shakti's call. Shakti's call is continuously present below the mind's chatter. It is the call of your divine nature, your bodhicitta, your Holy Spirit. Shakti speaks through silence, mantra, feelings, sensations, visions, synchronicities, symbols, urges, teachers and teachings, nature, and more. Learn her language, listen for her call, become intimately attuned to her.

Practice coming to rest in the heart, and see what opens your heart and draws you into deeper, more inclusive states of love. Explore what truly inspires you—art, music, creative expression, nature, choral music, temples, cathedrals, poetry. Whatever it might be, include it regularly in your daily or weekly practices.

Kundalini sadhana embraces Shakti's absolute authority with loving devotion, skill, discrimination, and surrender. It inspires us and requires us to serve others with love and compassion.

We have to develop discrimination to skillfully traverse this path. Study, contemplate, practice diligently, and interact with well informed, experienced, and trustworthy teachers and other students in order to further develop your discrimination. At all times keep good company. The practice of mental discipline is critical.

Kundalini unfolding is supported by practices of empowered mantra, Witness Consciousness, mindfulness, meditation, seva, chanting, hatha yoga, pranayama, the yamas and niyamas, cultivating positive attitudes towards yourself and others, aerobic exercise, and prana-filled food. By incorporating these into your everyday life, you will have a comprehensive set of sadhana practices.

Every moment gives us an opportunity for cultivating compassion, patience, kindness, and generosity. Every moment gives us an opportunity for cultivating an attitude of surrender: "Thy will be done."

14

Kriyas

Kundalini Recreating Mind and Body

Kriyas, the stirrings of awakened Kundalini, refer to movements of Shakti, the power of Consciousness actively recreating the mind and body. These are movements that clear and expand the capacities of the mind and body so they can more fully express the boundless love, compassion, wisdom, and creativity of your true Self. Kriyas further empower the mind and body to engage the processes of creating and reveling in the unfolding of life, taking on form, and consciously choosing limitations. Shakti didn't accidentally get caught in your form; She chose to be here as you. You are the Divine incarnate by choice; you've taken on limitations through your power to do so. But to know that and then to know that they're also reversible are the gifts of awakened Kundalini—your power of revelation and transformation. That's the kind of wisdom and freedom that we're invited to fully experience and directly know, not to just read about and love the idea of this state of radical freedom.

Kriyas are experienced in a staggeringly wide variety of ways, including inner lights, sounds, and visions; insights; profound wisdom; extraordinary creativity; wild rushes of emotion; complete stillness of mind; sensations of heat, electricity, or cold moving through the body; and shifts in awareness outside the body or outside the ordinary boundaries of time and space. Latent diseases, which are forms of karma, can be brought up and be dispelled or be embraced by our sadhana practices. Boundless love, compassion, and dissolution into Unity Consciousness are also kriyas. Yogic processes and practices can spontaneously manifest from kriyas. Kriyas can affect any organ system of the physical body and any capacity of the subtle body. Kundalini can move your consciousness, your mind, and your body in any way necessary to clear and expand the functioning of the mind-body system.

KRIYAS OF AWAKENING

People's experiences of awakening Kundalini are kriyas—Kundalini moving out of dormancy into action. Some people's experiences of this movement are very profound and dramatic, while others have experiences that are so subtle they can't even quite remember when awakening took place; they say something like, "All I know is over the last few years I've been transformed. Something must have happened when I started using the mantra and meditating because I'm happier and more loving." The kriyas that go with awakening can range from very subtle to very intense.

One individual who got in touch with me recently said he was just lying in bed doing a breathing exercise he learned in a hatha yoga class, and suddenly his body began writhing like a snake, arching up and down, and his breath began moving on its own, rapidly coming and going. His body suddenly went rigid, then completely still and almost lifeless, and his mind became absolutely blank. This was quite scary to him. He was not prepared for this experience; he didn't know what was going on and in trying to research what had happened to him, he found out about Kundalini. Those kinds of classic, dramatic physical kriyas can mark the beginning of the Kundalini awakening process.

For some people, Kundalini awakening might unfold with a vision or a dream, which are kriyas on a subtle body level when such events are the result of Shakti moving. One individual told me how he was on a shamanic vision quest some weeks before he was going to be working on Kundalini with me. On his vision quest, an extraordinary cobra appeared before him. The cobra seized his head in its mouth, and the flicking tongue of the cobra was touching his third eye, infusing him with energy. That marked his experience of shaktipat, awakening of Kundalini, which was followed by more profound and powerful experiences. This is another example of the classic form of Kundalini as a snake that many people have experienced in visions or dreams. That form can continue to present itself even after Kundalini awakening. People tell me about visitations they've had of snakes in their dreams bringing them gifts of wisdom, knowledge, insight, or influxes of energy. These are all subtle body kriyas, movements of Kundalini resulting in visions and dreams. As discussed in chapter 1, the image of the snake and the power of the snake to shed its skin and renew its life continue to be revered symbols of the Divine Feminine, especially in the Eastern traditions. She hasn't suffered the denigration that the snake symbol has in our Western patriarchal traditions. In the East, She continues to be a symbol of great wisdom and power and the gifts that come through the great goddess Kundalini.

KRIYAS OF KUNDALINI UNFOLDING

As Kundalini moves through the body and the mind in the course of sadhana, it creates many different kinds of changes and impacts our lives in countless ways. Some individuals experience extraordinary healing from psychological traumas, injuries to the body, physical diseases, joint troubles, allergies, cancer, mental illness, and more.

At the same time there are people, myself included, who have ailments that aren't healed. Some karmas have to be experienced; some are diminished and we are spared entirely from even knowing what they were. We don't get to choose which are which. As confusing and dismaying as this may be to the ego mind, Shakti doesn't go by a rule such as "heal everything needing to be healed." That's not what her purpose is. Her purpose is the transformation of the mind and body, the revelation of Unity Consciousness, and ultimately establishing one in a state of radical freedom, a state of Consciousness—not a body state, not a mind-born state, but the state of the Infinite. It may take more than one lifetime of work to burn up all the mind-body karmas we've accumulated that would have required millions of lifetimes to endure without the grace of awakened Kundalini.

I've experienced Shakti carrying me through extremely painful physical challenges—injuries, numerous surgeries, including three spinal surgeries, neuropathic pain, and more. Even in the midst of these physical challenges, Kundalini has moved my awareness into states of total ecstasy, of hearing sublime mantras emanating from the Infinite, even while crushing pain has wracked this body as it lay on a gurney in a hospital emergency room. The state of Kundalini, the state of the Self, transcends and includes all domains of awareness. This isn't a theory. This is my direct experience, and you are capable of knowing this truth for yourself. Many people have shared with me their experiences of having Shakti carry them through horrific traumas and near-death experiences. She will carry you through death itself and out the other side.

People consult me who have been through experiences of things happening with their body that when they first went to doctors, the doctors had absolutely no way of explaining them. Many have been to top clinics and hospitals in the country while having strange movements underneath their skin or anomalous bleeding in their body, all kinds of changes in fluids and muscles—muscles literally becoming decrepit and disappearing, then coming back—without any medical explanation. Even though doctors could observe the strange occurrences and noted them in the person's medical record, they couldn't explain them.

It turned out the experiences were all part of the process of Kundalini awakening and unfolding, unique to each particular individual. The actions of Kundalini transcend any model of Western medicine; they aren't bound by ordinary physical laws. And in fact, these kriyas, these movements of the power and energy of Kundalini, can impact any part of the entire range of what human experience includes. Anything that your body can experience can be moved and changed by Shakti—this is her vehicle, her creation—there are no limitations to how She can work on it to set you free.

USING DISCRIMINATION WITH KRIYAS

Developing discrimination is a fundamental component of understanding kriyas and how to receive what Kundalini is giving us through them. We need discrimination to be able to tell the difference between experience that's a kriya and experience that's our mind or our body. Is this happening because of a kriya or because there's something wrong with my endocrine system? Do I need a doctor or do I need a Kundalini guide to help me deal with what's going on right now?

I get email from people around the world who are going through various kinds of experiences, often difficult physical experiences that they may be attributing to Kundalini. At times it turns out to be something medical. My general advice for people is, when you have something going on physiologically, have it checked out by a physician. You'll want to rule out that there is some underlying physiological cause for what is going on with you that the mind may be mislabeling. I have seen cases where it did turn out to be an endocrinologic problem or some other medical condition, and the individual needed to have it addressed by their doctor.

If a person is having medical issues, it doesn't mean they aren't having Kundalini experiences in addition to that. Sometimes dealing with health challenges is an awakening and has profound spiritual lessons for a person. But the physiological disorder or disease has to be dealt with effectively.

EGO MIND: LET GO AND LET SHAKTI

The ego can react to the types of kriyas that are possible as if it entered the ultimate candy store for the mind! Shakti's kriyas include the entire range of what your mind can experience, from the subtlest of emotions to the wildest of visions, to the most profound dreams, to the depths of despair, and on up to super-sensuous ecstasy. Shakti may bestow any kind of experience—profound insights, intuition, powers of clairvoyance or clairaudience, all of these are all her possible creations. She can work with them at any time and in any way. She doesn't do it systematically from our mind's limited view. That's often a misunderstanding that people carry over from the system of chakras. The chakra map provides a theoretical model for understanding how Kundalini Shakti moves through these centers of consciousness that She has created. But it's not an elevator. It's a mistake to think Kundalini is going to go through level by level in a simplistic way. The ego mind loves the illusion of prediction and control and how that illusion supports its fantasies of getting kriyas it wants. It's good to let go of that and simply be present in the moment with one's sadhana and practices.

Some people have tried to do a systematic approach using their ego mind to direct Kundalini. There are books written with instructions to move your Kundalini here, move your awareness from one chakra to the other, and so forth. But it gets people caught in the illusion that it's actually the way it's going to work when, in fact, the great goddess Kundalini is running the show, not the ego mind. The ego mind is so attached to its fantasy of being in charge, of being the one controlling the process, that it is petrified to discover it is not. Watch what happens to ego mind in death. The Tibetan Buddhist teachings on the *bardo* (the transitional state between lives) are important for understanding what happens to the ego mind when confronted with huge energies beyond its control and comprehension. Chögyam Trungpa Rinpoche's teachings on this are particularly lucid.

The mind can move prana with powerful effects that can be similar to some of Kundalini's effects, but without Kundalini's wisdom. Many people have told me of their experiences of serious pranic disturbances caused by the unskillful use of yogic and meditative practices. Kundalini is the source and prime mover of prana. Kundalini will let the ego live out that drama and the karmas it creates playing in the limited sandbox of the mind for lifetimes if necessary. To get to radical freedom, it's better for the ego mind to let go of its intense desire to be in charge. It has to let go of seeking particular experiences or powers it desires. The mind can invite Kundalini to move to an area needing healing or release. The mind can pray to Kundalini for the strength and wisdom it needs to move through a difficulty. Know this: Kundalini moves only because She chooses to. Her movements are filled with grace. To fully receive her grace, we need to let go of the ego and all its illusions of being the doer.

There's a part of us that knows that it takes more than visualizations and exercises to fully, consciously enter the subtle body, Kundalini's creation. If you visualize the Grand Canyon, even if you've seen pictures of the Grand Canyon and how magnificent it is in all its colors and if you visualized it very clearly, over and over, it would be nothing compared to the direct experience of going to the Grand Canyon and standing on the edge, seeing that mind-boggling, mile-deep opening in the earth. The best visualization is nothing compared to the real thing. So on one level, we know that merely visualizing something isn't the same as the direct experience. Yet, when we go into these spiritual realms, we lose the common sense wisdom that we already have.

The direct experience of going into the chakras and into these archetypal levels of human consciousness, being drawn there by Kundalini, is entirely different than visualizing them and convincing ourselves that just by visualizing them, we've actually made them happen. Visualization techniques can be useful and can help prime the mind and body for opening to certain experiences, but they're not the same as the full-blown direct gift of that experience that comes through Kundalini Shakti. Yogis, for thousands of years, have done extraordinary practices, some taking a lifetime to master, in order to directly know the subtle body, awaken Kundalini, and be pulled by her grace through the transformation of all the chakras. If it were as easy as visualizing it, they wouldn't go to that effort. Kundalini will allow one to roam the mirror-maze of the mind's delusions for as long as one wants. Better to invoke her aid with love and surrender to her direction.

There are physical kriyas that can move the body in a variety of ways, shaking the body, causing different sensations that move through the body—heat, electricity, fire, ice, water, air—and even going into spontaneous hatha yoga postures. These movements are known to other traditions as well. For example in the Christian tradition, Quakers experience some of these same things as the Holy Spirit moves through them, making them quake or shake. People who've never done any hatha yoga may find themselves automatically doing asanas, pranayamas, mudras, bandhas, and more. I've seen people go into spontaneous headstands and do spontaneous mudras (hand movements that move and seal in energy). People have these happen effortlessly though they had absolutely no prior experience of them. All these kriyas occur by the power of Kundalini moving through the subtle body, the mind, and the physical body. Often they are accompanied by experiences of bliss and energy or of the mind going into Witness Consciousness. At other times, the mind might wander or be caught in thought even while Shakti is doing her miraculous work.

Some of the most challenging kriyas are ones impacting the mind, because we are so identified with our mind and the content of our mind—the thoughts, feelings, sensations, memories, and so forth. When that inner world is shaken by Shakti, it really rattles us—our very sense of self can be challenged. Some of these experiences can feel very destabilizing. The mind can race, emotions can fluctuate wildly, and there can be descents into the dark corners of our unconscious that we'd rather never face. But Kundalini is Consciousness; She goes everywhere; She illumines everything and is one-pointed in her intention to set us free.

This cleansing process can also challenge our belief structures and create profound changes in them. As I mentioned in chapter 3, my doctoral research showed the transformative process of Kundalini encompassed everything. Every aspect of the subjects' lives would change, including beliefs as fundamental as those defining who they are, what the nature of a human being is, and what the meaning and purpose of life is. When Kundalini Shakti is revealing and giving you the direct experience that you are Divine, that all others are Divine, that this world is an unfolding of divinity moment by moment, that we are all connected and united as One, then how could it not change your beliefs? How could it not transform how you relate to yourself, others, and the world around you? This can be challenging for the ego mind that has based its identity on old patterns for its entire life, so it may struggle to deal with these things. It needs patience, compassion, and support to adjust to such radical changes. It may also need professional help from a transpersonal psychologist to integrate these kinds of life altering changes.

LETTING GO OF DISTRACTIONS

All kriyas, regardless of how they are impacting the body or impressing the mind with the power and glory of what Shakti creates, can become distractions if the mind gets involved. This is why Witness Consciousness and mindfulness are such important foundational practices. No matter how mundane or extraordinary kriyas may appear to the ordinary mind, watch them with the detached awareness of the Witness. Kriyas can be so numinous, so alluring and seductive that the mind can get deluded and lost in them for very long periods of time. For this reason, many spiritual traditions advise practitioners to ignore them completely, even suppress them, in order not to get side-tracked by them. In the Christian tradition, Saint Teresa of Avila called the movements of the Holy Spirit that she experienced *consolations*. They were the consolations that God gives along the spiritual path, not to be confused with the great gift of grace—union with the Divine.

The very nature of our sense of self begins to change under Kundalini's beneficent influence, and part of what helps to ease that process is to give the ego mind a refuge. It can have its own place, its own identity, but no longer as the master, the dominator of your inner worlds busily trying to organize the universe to fulfill its desires. That old egocentric perspective will no longer serve. Now the ego mind is given the sacred place of the servant. The ego mind doesn't have to try to become the Infinite Self, though it usually does try! But if it does, it will become inflated, it will become dysfunctional and even more deluded. The ego mind's job is focused on the answers to the questions: How do I serve in this moment? How do I serve the Divine Self, present in everyone at all times? How do I do this with the loving care, devotion, skills, knowledge, and capabilities that I've been given to serve with? By reorienting the ego mind moment by moment to selflessly serve through fulfilling its dharma, it becomes the servant of love and compassion, attuned to the Divine.

The path of Kundalini, the path of knowing and serving the Divine Presence, is always the path of shifting from "my will be done" to "thy will be done." That shift is an extraordinarily profound transformation for the ego mind because it has spent its entire life trying to figure out how to get its will to be done. Now it has to transform that into discriminating, knowing, intuiting, and following the unfolding power of grace in our own inner world as well as the world around us. This is not a rational endeavor, and the rational mind can be severely challenged by Kundalini sadhana.

The path of Kundalini is one of increasing awareness of Shakti's guidance. Because the Divine isn't typically speaking in a loud, clear voice telling us what we should do, the ego mind has to develop subtle discrimination to free itself of what allures it unconsciously. While developing discrimination and surrendering to the highest, the ego mind is given practices such as the yamas and niyamas, the Noble Eightfold Path, bodhisattva vows, and so forth that guide and contain the ego mind's actions until it has become completely attuned to ways of compassion, love, kindness, and patience.

Many people cut to the quick and ask, "How do I follow Kundalini?" Here's how to start: begin with deepening and expanding the practices in the yamas and niyamas, along with other practices such as empowered mantra, meditation, and seva. The yamas and niyamas provide concrete steps that you can do in everyday life that will transform and contain the ego mind. Adherence to the yamas and niyamas is a practical way of containing the ego mind and reducing the moment-by-moment disruptions to sadhana it creates, as well as reducing the long-term karmas it produces, which will take lifetimes to work through. Shakti, the living presence of Kundalini within you, will help guide you. Additionally, having the support of one who truly knows the ways of Kundalini, as hard as they are to find, is of incalculable benefit. There are people like myself who guide individuals and give empowered practices to support them on their path. I can't imagine what abyss I'd be lost in without the support of my teachers and Shakti herself.

Buddha gave us the Noble Eightfold Path twenty-five hundred years ago as an extraordinary guide to sadhana. It provides for awakening to the truth of who you are, as well as for grounding and integrating full wakefulness into everyday life. It was given at the same time that the eight limbs of yoga were practiced and taught through an oral tradition. If you study Buddha's Noble Eightfold Path, you will see that it is another structured set of practices for transforming the ego mind and awakening you to your innate nature, your Buddha mind. It is another path for following Kundalini, and some of the Tibetan Buddhist rinpoches I've met speak about Kundalini as one of the most esoteric and closely held set of teachings in their traditions.

Just as in the yogic tradition, the Noble Eightfold Path recognizes avidya, primal ignorance, and the constantly craving ego mind that springs from it as the sources of suffering. The fully awakened mind, your Buddha mind, is the innate source of the radical freedom you come to know by extinguishing attachment to and identification with the ephemeral ego mind. The Noble Eightfold Path includes practices for developing wisdom, practices for developing ethics, and practices for developing and deepening meditation. All together they form a sacred container, giving the ego mind a way to be grounded in service and compassionately engaged, while at the same time you're cultivating the experience of infinite spaciousness of awareness, the true nature of your Buddha mind, your bodhicitta, free of the conditioned mind, free of the root of suffering.

WITNESSING KRIYAS

Kundalini empowers you to be detached, able to watch and encourage the ego mind. The spontaneous arising of the wise and compassionate Witness, the inner guru/guide, is a profound kriya, a movement and bestowal of grace by Shakti. The ego is going to struggle with the practices and the kriyas; it's going to resist training. That's tapasya, and it is a natural part of sadhana. The mind can be like an undisciplined dog that has run wild, and now you are putting it on a very short leash. It will react. You learn to see where and when you can let it run and when to reel it in. The ego mind needs the inner presence that has the compassion and the patience to work with it, to re-form it in the mold of a loving, kind, compassionate, energetic, creative, and skillful servant of your highest nature. That's what happens by following these disciplines under the guidance of a compassionate mentor. Kundalini is the reflective power, the illuminating power of Witness Consciousness, the Self, and can guide the mind when the mind becomes clear enough and steady enough to receive that guidance without distortion. The ego mind plays its game for a long time! That's why serious yoga and meditation students always need an outside reference point—the clear, disciplined consciousness of a trustworthy and selfless teacher, and an informed and dedicated sangha, the community of practitioners.

Right now many people in desperation are seeking guidance from others who have little knowledge and experience and who never were properly mentored or taught themselves. Even with good intentions, this is only the blind leading the blind, exchanging half-truths and delusions, prolonging suffering. The Internet amplifies this. There's no discrimination filter on the Internet. You have to bring that to your studies, to your review of resources that you might access. Cultivate viveka and avoid the uninformed. An uninformed opinion is worth what you pay for it. But following it can cost you years, if not lifetimes, of effort.

CULTIVATING STEADY AWARENESS

Kriyas are movements of Shakti that produce visions, emotions, insights, sounds, bodily movements and sensations, and more. These are all simply movements of energy. This is also true of the ordinary movements of our mind and body that we are familiar with and think nothing of. Cultivating steady awareness in the face of movement, regardless of whether the source is Shakti, the mind, or the body, is essential in sadhana.

Sit in your best meditation posture, withdraw your attention from the outer world, closing your eyes and allowing your mind to follow the movements of your breath. Invite the breath to slow and deepen, inviting the body to let go and settle more and more deeply with each breath.

Notice that there is a very brief pause between the inhalation and the exhalation, between the exhalation and the inhalation. There is an instant of stillness between the breaths. The movements of the breath arise out of stillness and dissolve into stillness. Watch for the stillness. Shift your attention away from movement and watch for the stillness.

Now shift your attention to the mind, the thoughts and sensations, the memories and feelings, the images and perceptions that come and go through the mind. Between these movements there is stillness. Look for the stillness between the thought waves. Shift your attention away from the movements of the mind and notice the stillness between the thoughts. As you focus more on the stillness that is unmoved by movements of the mind or body, your awareness will grow steadier, stronger, and become unshakeable by whatever happens.

15

Challenges on the Path

When people say that Kundalini sadhana is challenging or that there are many obstacles and distractions, it is worth inquiring about who is being challenged or obstructed. Who gets distracted? It certainly isn't the Self, or Kundalini. It isn't your Buddha mind or Christ consciousness. Rather, it is the ego mind that experiences challenges, gets lost in distractions, is seduced by sideshows and becomes fearful, irritable, or overwhelmed. It is the ego mind that wanders off the path in the pursuit of power or some other nugget of fool's gold it finds on the path. Remember that the ego mind is always trying to negotiate the world by seeking what it believes will be most pleasurable and avoiding what appears painful. It brings that conditioned set of responses to spiritual pursuits as well, with or without Kundalini awakening. Even when the ego mind's pleasure-seeking is refined, this is a superficial level of existence.

Each and every human being has a much, much deeper level of existence that is unfolding through the course of their life. That's our soul's journey; that's Kundalini or Holy Spirit, calling us home, guiding our life in profound ways whether we're in the savritti phase or the nivritti phase. As that power of Consciousness awakens at a deeper level, bringing to awareness the importance of a precious human birth with the possibility of evolving through this lifetime, connecting with the Divine essence at our core becomes a prime motivator. We can't squander this precious birth by continuing to be driven by our old mammalian and reptilian brains! Once awakening illumines our life with the wisdom, the boundless compassion, and the infinite love that we have the capacity to bring into this world through our mindful attention, then our actions, our attitudes, our pursuits, and everything changes. The ego mind is empowered to serve the sublime impulses arising from our highest Self instead of the conditioned mind-brain.

MIND-BORN CHALLENGES

Most of the challenges on the spiritual path are generated by the ego mind. As I said earlier, virtually all the practices of yoga, meditation, prayer, chanting, vipassana, mindfulness, visualizations, mantra, yantra, tantra, ritual, and on and on are all for the mind and body. They aim at strengthening and healing the body, transforming the mind, clearing the mind, stabilizing the mind, deconstructing the ego, and freeing one from samskaras and karmas. The Infinite reveals what lies beyond the conditioned mind—the already fully present Unity Consciousness. Your fully awakened Self, your fully realized Buddha mind, your unconditionally loving Christ consciousness already exists and needs no work, no self-help courses!

The doing mind, the ego mind, is challenged by wanting to do and do and do, as it always does, in order to produce and possess this enlightenment, this radical freedom, this nirvana, this state of extinguished craving. The ego mind can't "do" it. It's like one trying to jump over one's shadow. Eventually it exhausts itself, and in the ensuing stillness, it experiences some of the radiance of the ever-present Infinitude, only to jump up, break the stillness, and go running after another mirage. Every seeker goes through this. Every master has been through this. Every master has watched their students go through this, day after day, week after week, month after month, year after year, lifetime after lifetime. Better to breathe and let go right now! Discrimination is the power of discernment that you cultivate in order to see the ego mind and what it creates. Discrimination also empowers you to discern the ways that Kundalini is inviting you to get free from the ego mind's patterns.

In the course of sadhana, we inform the mind through practices, study, contemplation, and selfless service. We keep the mind and body occupied with these things while the power of grace, Kundalini, does the multiple levels of transformative work that the mind and body simply cannot do. Of course the ego mind is very impressed with its own efforts! It will shed endless drops of sweat doing asanas, believing in the importance of its efforts, until it encounters Kundalini, true awakening. All the limbs of yoga are beneficial for the mind and body to practice. And it is humbling for the ego mind to experience that in one moment of Kundalini's blazing energy; She will accomplish what lifetimes of yoga practice attempts.

In the ancient Indian Ayurvedic system of medicine, dis-ease results from one of three sources: what you think, what you eat, and karma. Kundalini and yoga sadhana practices aim at transforming the mind and what you feed it, transforming the body and what you feed it as well, and ameliorating the karmic challenges we face from past actions. Kundalini awakening and unfolding are prized because they free the seeker from mountains of karma that would otherwise take countless lifetimes to eradicate. She's doing it on levels where the ego mind isn't even aware of it. At the same time, the experiences one is going through can feel very challenging at times. The ordinary ego mind might even blame Kundalini for the pain it is going through. Discrimination allows us to see through the reactivity of the mind and body and stay steady with our practices, remaining aligned with Kundalini's energies of transformation.

Some people tell me Kundalini is doing the wrong thing (as if their ego mind knows better than Universal Consciousness); Kundalini is making them so uncomfortable; Kundalini is giving them so much pain; they wish Kundalini would stop and go away forever. These sentiments are understandable from the viewpoint of the ego mind. It doesn't want to face the consequences of its own karmas, its own actions, its own patterns that have been laid down over lifetimes. But in fact, the grace of Kundalini is working to free it from all that, and whether those experiences are painful or ecstatic, expansive or contracted, delightful or difficult, they're all related to what has to be cleared, what has to be opened, what has to be transformed through the grace of Kundalini. It's important to cultivate that understanding so we can go through the difficult times and understand we can celebrate that we're being freed of whatever those patterns are. We can practice an uplifting attitude. We may not even know what the roots of that painful experience are, but we can celebrate that we are getting free of it and that we are being moved through it by divine grace. We can take hold of the kinds of practices that give us the steadiness and strength for moving through the challenges as gracefully as we can, with support from those we love, the practices, and our teachers and mentors. A teacher can help you assess what changes in practices or additional practices may be needed to ease Kundalini's work through the blockages and the karmas that need to be cleared.

I never hear people complain about the ecstatic experiences, but they do complain that they don't stay the same, or their favorite one hasn't repeated itself, or the beginning of Kundalini unfolding was like a honeymoon, but now it's just drudgery! The ego mind will always have things to complain about until it is at last free to stay in the presence of the Divine, ready to serve. Then its delight becomes continuous. The ego mind is locked in the domain of attraction and aversion, pleasure and pain. Over time, through strengths developed by the practices and by the grace of your own Self, you learn not to take the ego mind too seriously. You look at it with discrimination, sifting what is important for sadhana from what isn't.

One of the main developments that occurs over time with the unfolding of Kundalini is that we gain greater and greater ability to discern Shakti's call, the directions in which Shakti wants to move your sadhana, through everything from daily practices to life decisions. There are foundational practices such as daily meditation, daily practice of mantra, seva, exercise, and hatha yoga, which keep the mind and body clear and aligned. But there may be other times when specific practices are called for, specific contemplations, less meditation or more meditation, fewer asanas or more asanas, more chanting or less, studying and contemplating specific texts, dietary changes, or changes in relationships, and the list goes on.

In the course of sadhana, we have to bring our discrimination to bear on our relationships, seeing which relationships are energy drains that need to be changed or relinquished, and which have more energy and power to support sadhana and growth. This kind of discernment, or discrimination, is necessary for traversing the path of Kundalini. It is incumbent upon the seeker to listen more and more deeply, more and more profoundly, for what Shakti is calling you to do, to be aware of her directions and how to shift and move with her dance, her play, her path that's unfolding beneath your feet.

Kundalini sadhana encompasses all of life, all activities, and all moments. Within this broad context, there are several typical challenge areas people encounter that can be like the turbulent rapids and waterfalls on a river. The river will carry you to the sea, but you need to know how to navigate the river of Shakti in order to make it to the ocean of the Divine without falling overboard! We'll look at the major areas that need careful attention: fear and anger, integrating high energy and staying grounded, traumatic life experiences, and chronic illness. This isn't an exhaustive list. You may have areas that are uniquely challenging for you, and you may want to gain support and guidance to skillfully navigate them.

FEAR AND ANGER

There are certain challenges that are particularly provocative for Kundalini processes. Just as Kundalini works to clear the body of blocks and perhaps latent diseases that prevent the body from fully participating in the joy of knowing the Infinite and manifesting that in everyday life, Kundalini also works throughout the mind, on both conscious and unconscious levels. All of us carry in our bodies and in our minds conditioned responses. Two in particular trigger a lot of problems for people, in spiritual practice in general, but in particular with the energy of Kundalini, and these are fear and anger.

Fear is seen from a yogic perspective as something that's rooted in the primal ignorance, avidya, which I discussed earlier. It's the ignorance of not knowing who and what we truly are. That ignorance is the foundation for the ego, and fear is something that is as much a part of the untransformed ego as all of its limitations. It fears losing what it thinks it is attached to or possesses, and it fears not getting what it desperately wants. The ego can be fearful of things that are greater than it, stronger than it, separate, and different from it. Being a separate individual is a basic quality of avidya-created ego. In the1986 hit "All Around The World or The Myth of Fingerprints," Paul Simon sung about this, "It was the myth of fingerprints, that's why we must learn to live alone."[1] The illusion of being completely separate, unique individuals is why we inflict so much pain on others and have endless wars. When fear is triggered, it also triggers aspects of our neurophysiological instrument, the brain-body. These drive irrational behaviors. These easily triggered fear reactions also can cause people to feel very stressed by Kundalini's energies moving through their systems. Their fight-flight-freeze stress response is activated, releasing adrenaline and other stress hormones into the mind-brain-body system. Deep relaxation skills, slow diaphragmatic breathing, Witness meditation, and mindfulness training are good for down-regulating the autonomic nervous system's stress response. Biofeedback and neurofeedback training can be very beneficial.

Anger can also trigger many of the same fight-flight-freeze responses of the autonomic nervous system. Anger is closely related to fear as another quality of the conditioned ego mind that is rooted in avidya, the primal ignorance that blocks our awareness of our inherent fullness of Being. Believing ourselves to be limited creates the experience of lack and want. Because the ego mind by the nature of its limitations thinks it has some things, thinks it doesn't have other things, and wants things that it doesn't have, when it doesn't get them, it provokes frustration, irritability, and anger. The ego mind, which is incomplete and lacking so many things, is subject to being triggered all the time by anger and fear. It becomes irritated and angry when it doesn't get what it wants, and it becomes fearful of losing things that it clings to.

The ego is the power of self-appropriation. It appropriates things to itself that it likes and wants even if it has to possess them by identifying with them. The ego goes through life taking hold of things—you could be driving down the road, and suddenly the ego mind owns the road, "They just pulled into my lane!" People have road rage, parking lot rage, and even Christmas shopping rage that turns deadly! This is an entirely out-of-control ego mind. But the reactivity is also a part of the nervous system that's being triggered. Energetically, Kundalini can be very difficult for people when they carry those kinds of samskaras—patterns of reactivity, of easily triggered irritability, anger, and fear. People often discover that it seems as if Kundalini is amplifying those things, and they feel powerful surges of energy in their body or their mind. They feel like their emotions are getting out of control as Kundalini is working to clear these patterns of reactivity out of the body-mind complex.

What we have to do if we're going through that process is expand the container, expand the mind's capacity for sitting in, tolerating, and being present with those experiences without being compelled to act on them. This gives us the freedom to watch with greater and greater equanimity as Shakti clears out whatever the stuck pattern might be without the mind becoming overwhelmed. That's part of what I talked about at the end of chapter 5 in terms of practicing Witness Consciousness, mindfulness training, and vipassana meditation. They involve stepping back from the mind-body activity and letting go. Stepping back and not identifying with every thought or feeling or thing that moves through the mind, stepping back from those patterns whether they are fear-based or anger-based, and then simply breathing and letting go. Meet each reaction with a state that's relaxed, detached, aware—neither pushing it down nor identifying with it. That expands the container and allows the fluidity of energy to move through and clear these things. One of my early teachers, Chögyam Trungpa Rinpoche, would speak about giving the wild and restless cow of the mind a large meadow in which to play and expend its energy as you tame it. Then it quiets down without one having to expend so much energy fighting to restrain it. You separate yourself from the mind, and this gives you new choices. If the mind goes crazy, choose not to go with it! This isn't easy at first, but you will delight in the mastery you develop with practice. Buddha said, "Whoever doesn't flare up at someone who is angry wins a battle hard to win."[2]

Shakti frees us of patterns of reactivity and anger on many different levels. I mentioned earlier that I had done volunteer work teaching meditative practices in prisons. An incident happened at a program I ran in a federal penitentiary that highlights the kinds of transformations that occur with Kundalini awakening. There was a fellow who was coming to the regular weekly meditation program that focused on the use of mantra for meditation and japa—the practice of repeating the mantra whenever the mind isn't engaged in a necessary task. Mantra is one of the most powerful vehicles for conveying awakened Kundalini, and I certainly saw its power while working in prisons.

This inmate was coming pretty regularly, and he was a very angry individual. He had been in prison for fifteen to eighteen years of a thirty-five year sentence. He had a history of a lot of angry acting-out that prevented him from getting paroled. I had been warned by one of the prison staff that he often had angry encounters with guards, and in prison there's a very antagonistic dynamic between these two groups. In fact, the program that we held was barely supported by the prison. We were given a dirty lounge room to hold the meditation program in, and at the back of that room there were vending machines. Invariably the guards would come in to use the vending machines while we were in the midst of a program or a meditation, just to disrupt things because something nice was being done for inmates. The guards would come in simply to interfere with it. That was just a sad fact of how those cultures interacted.

One night while holding the program, we were chanting Om Namah Shivaya, and during the chant, sure enough, one of the guards came in, went to the back of the room and loudly slammed his quarters into the soda machine. The soda machine clunked and dropped its can of Pepsi—but here a very unusual thing happened. The guard got his can of soda and then sat down in the back of the room. Guards never join in inmate activities, it just never happens. And in all the programs I've done in prisons, more than 150 of them, a guard has never stayed around. So something unusual was happening. We continued the chant, went into the meditation, and the guard still sat there through the whole meditation. This never happens. At the end of the meditation we did a few rounds of the chant Om Namah Shivaya upon coming out of meditation, and as it ended the guard got up and started to leave.

In that moment, the inmate who has a history of being very angry and acting out also got up to leave. I saw him striding toward the guard. I was playing the harmonium, finishing the chant, just watching and wondering what was going to happen. They exchanged a few words in the back of the room, the guard left, and the inmate came back and sat down. We finished up the program. Sometimes at the end guys would say a few words, but typically not. Prison is not a touchy feely place; you don't share what's going on inside of you. But interestingly this inmate said, "You know, I have to say something. I had a run-in with that guard in the yard today; I was really furious with him. And I said some things and carried that anger away with me even as I left the yard. And then tonight, we're sitting there, we're doing this chant, we're doing the meditation, and that guy comes in, and something changed. So at the end of the meditation, I felt like I had to get up," and he said, "I had to apologize to him!" He again said, "I had to apologize!"

He was incredulous. He was a little sheepish about even saying it, because you don't want to admit vulnerability or weakness in front of other inmates either—that's not a cool thing. But he was saying this in front of other guys. He said, "I can't believe it; I felt like I had to apologize to the guard!" And then he said, "The strangest thing was, then the guard said, 'you know, I don't know what you guys were doing in here. I came in here just to get a soda and get out of here and that chant you were doing, it just moved me somehow. I had to sit down. And then, that period of silence afterward felt so good. I felt so good.' He said, 'just something changed.'" And the two of them had a completely different interaction than they ever would have had before.

When I speak about Kundalini transforming the mind, freeing it of patterns of anger, reactivity, and conditioning, patterns that bind the mind to reacting and acting over and over again in the same ways, repeatedly creating the same kinds of suffering that we experience, it is this kind of profound transformation that I'm referring to. The inmate had been trapped in a lifelong pattern of actions, and the guard was caught in his own patterns as well as prison-culture ways of interacting. When those two individuals could be free in that moment, then you see the power of Shakti, the power of mantra and practice. Both were freed to step out of bondage so they could experience each other and life in a different way. This is how Kundalini Shakti transforms everyday life. They didn't have to have visions of divine lights coming and settling on their head, or anything like that—that's not what it's about. This is an example of a very grounded, integrated, in-the-moment freedom to experience life in a different way. That's what it is to step out of the normal ways that our mind creates our reality and our patterns of relating and interacting with the world. This is Kundalini's gift; this is how She transforms our experience.

It's good for us to contemplate what goes on in our own mind, what imprisons us, what binds us in a situation: what is my mind stuck identifying with in this moment? By being able to look at things this way, we begin to be more mindful of what's going on in our consciousness and what those patterns are. How do we step out of them? Even if Kundalini is inviting us to be free of patterns, the ego mind has to participate in that transformation and cultivate new and different patterns of being in the world and acting in the world. It has to risk doing things differently, and it has to learn how to do things differently. Learning to do things differently can involve taking skills training such as assertiveness, anger management, stress mastery, parenting, coaching, or whatever you need. These too become part of one's sadhana practices.

Working with the ego mind in a contained and contemplative way means really seeing what happens when anger arises in you. Anger binds people. Anger is an emotion that's very difficult for people to contain and deal with in an effective way. Most spiritual disciplines focus on the absolute level of getting completely free of anger so there's no danger of acting on it.

Being completely free of any pressure to act on anger is essential. Once that is achieved, then we can view anger and examine it. Stepping back from anger and being able to see the power of the anger in the moment, ask yourself, what's the energy of the anger directed at? Anger is an energy that in the moment says, "I don't like what's going on. Here is a bundle of energy, something needs to change, create something different." In a way, that is the hidden wisdom of anger. There's energy being made available to create change. Most of the time, people don't have the container to wisely view anger and harness its energy. They just blow the energy out, shooting off their mouth or doing something angrily. It doesn't really create change; it creates more negativity. Or people just repress it, and that has its negative consequences as well.

The strong container, like a gold crucible that is built through the workings of Kundalini, mantra, meditation, and contemplation, allows us to hold the powerful energies that need to be transmuted. Having that container allows us to be detached and aware of the energy of anger, a reaction that basically says, "Something's wrong here; something needs to change; here's some energy to change it." With practice, we bring the light of awareness to the moment, knowing that our container can hold that energy without automatically spilling it everywhere. We can look at anger and consider what needs to change? Does something need to change inside? Maybe it's my attitude; maybe it's my approach; maybe it's my way of viewing the situation. Or does something need to change outside? Maybe it's the situation or another person's behavior, or some combination of both that needs to change. Then we're in the spacious and free place of awareness to be able to take hold of that energy and say, "Now, how do I use this energy in the best way possible to serve the highest in this moment, to create change in the most skillful way possible?" Your wisdom, your insight, transforms the situation. Anger, instead of being an emotion that takes hold of you and possesses you, becomes a power, Shakti, a creative force for positive change. What you do with that energy won't look like anger at all; it will take the form of wisdom, creativity, and compassion. You can develop the capacity to recognize that you have this energy called "anger," that you can reflect on it and use it creatively to make changes in an effective manner. You have the freedom to ask yourself: What will I do with this energy? How do I use it in a way to create the change that needs to happen? How can I effect the changes that need to happen internally, externally, or both? And how can I do this in a way that's skillful, compassionate, and nonviolent? That's the kind of freedom and spaciousness of awareness that awakened Shakti Kundalini gives us when combined with the self-discipline of practice. It's the reflective space that the power of Consciousness and the practices start to provide us, the sacred container that holds the mind, empowering us to step back from volatile emotions like anger and transform them. This transforms the impact they have on us and on everyone around us.

Your true nature, your Buddha nature, your Divine Self, is free of the automatic reactivity of the mind. The more Shakti pulls you into states that give you access to your innate wisdom, the more the ordinary mind is deconditioned and freed from reactivity. We practice restraint while there's still something to restrain. When wisdom permeates the mind, there's nothing left to restrain. That's radical freedom.

Everyone has triggers to begin with—things that set them off, things that they are sensitive to, or things that come up when they are very tired or haven't eaten or are stressed out. Some retreat practices are specifically designed to exhaust and sleep-deprive the ego mind so it can't summon the strength to posture steady wisdom, deep compassion, profound patience, or true freedom. The ego mind can be quite accomplished at such posturing until a trigger reveals its deception. To be radically free, to have Kundalini complete her work, you have to get completely clear of all triggers, all the things that the mind would ordinarily react to with anger or irritability, impatience or loss of equanimity and compassion. Praise and blame are emblematic of such triggers that the ego mind is afflicted by. Shakti confronts us with how we react to praise, what part of the mind loves it, seeks it, is conditioned to go after it. What part of us reacts to blame and shame, when we're told negative things, given negative feedback, criticized, or treated disrespectfully? She demands that we see the ego mind and its limitations and afflictions. Freedom requires going beyond the qualities of attraction and aversion, in all their forms. Shakti can create circumstances in our lives that confront us with our shortcomings, with how the ego mind plays out these dramas of seeking praise, avoiding blame, or other forms of conditioning the mind is caught in. Skillful use of the mindfulness practices and mantra, Witness Consciousness, and taking refuge in the Self frees the mind from its samskaras.

LETTING GO OF THE EGO MIND, MERGING WITH "I AM"

Kundalini opens a person's awareness to the nature of the ego mind, with all its limitations and afflictions, while at the same time opening their consciousness to the boundless nature of their true Self, the Infinite One. Seeing the ego mind from the vantage point of the Self, through the eyes of Kundalini, shifts the ego out of a place of dominance. Then as Kundalini continues to unfold and one engages in sadhana practices such as the self-discipline required for following the Noble Eightfold Path or Classical yoga, the ego is transformed. At the same time one gains freedom from having it monopolize consciousness. As Kundalini repeatedly draws a person's consciousness into transcendent states and union with the Infinite, the limited I-awareness of the ego mind no longer is the only state of consciousness discernable. These experiences further develop one's discrimination. Spontaneous experiences of transcendence and union, in addition to the ones that occur through meditative practices, are essential for transforming the ego and freeing one's consciousness from its confines. Since anger and fear arise from the limited and wanting nature of the ego, the real antidote is direct knowledge and experience of the Self.

Central to the practice of Witness Consciousness is the process of merger and identification with the Self or with its vibratory equivalent—mantra. Letting go of the ego mind and all it identifies with is part of that process. This complements the ego transformation work that is done through other yogic practices. By stepping back and letting go, entering meditation by letting go of the ego, the mind, and all you usually identify with, your consciousness comes to rest in the unconditioned awareness of "I Am," the pure I-am awareness free of all conditioning, free of I am happy, sad, thinking, reacting . . . That pure I-am awareness may arise from merging with the mantra. I am Om Kali Ma, I am a throb of the Infinite, or I am Hamsa, the throb of I-am awareness whispered with every breath. Hamsa is the ancient mantra of the Self as the breath comes in with *Hammm* and goes out with *Saaa*. Merge in that and know the Self.

HAMSA

My Dear One,
You've sought to see me
as you wanted to see me.

You've sought to hold me
as you wanted to hold me.

You've caught glimpses of your Beloved
and your eyes filled with tears of joy
washing away the suffering of the world.

You've felt the brush of my Holy Spirit
and delighted in the ecstasy
that blossomed in your body.

My Dear One,
It is time to
surrender.

Surrender seeking to see me
as you want to see me.

Surrender seeking to hold me
as you want to hold me.

It is time to behold me as

I Am.

KALIDAS[3]

INTEGRATING KUNDALINI'S ENERGIES OF TRANSFORMATION

One liberating insight that Kundalini provides is the way in which the mind and body are vehicles of Shakti's creation for exploring and experiencing our everyday life, the world of forms, the world that we know of relationships, of our families, and our work. It's by solely identifying with these vehicles, the vehicles of the mind and body, that we become them and suffer their limitations. The insight that Kundalini, our inner Light of Consciousness, gives us is the realization that the vehicles of the mind and body are our creations that we've poured our awareness into by identifying with them, by saying in essence "I am this mind, I am this body, I am a man" or "I am a woman, I am young, I am old, I am fat, I am happy, I am sad." Moment by moment the psychic instrument of the ego identifies with thoughts, feelings, memories, roles, and so on. As we identify with whatever state that vehicle is in, we then fully experience it. That's the dynamic of how consciousness gets to experience limitation. This is not an accident or a mistake. This is how Infinite Universal Consciousness explores the experience of limited consciousness.

We are organs of experience for the Infinite Divine. You are the organ of the Infinite for knowing Itself in the beautiful form of you, knowing your life as it is, as a creation of the Divine creator. This is not a mistake. You are experiencing it because you are the eyes, the ears, the nose, the skin, the mouth, everything for the Divine experiencing the course of your life as it is. Kundalini invites you to join in the awareness of the grandeur underlying this experience, of the Infinite knowledge and delight that your true Self experiences in the midst of your finite experience.

Kundalini empowers your limited consciousness to step back and say, "Oh, that's what's going on! This is the dynamic! Not only do I have this individual experience, I can also have simultaneously the universal experience and with that have my individual self informed by that greater wisdom." Shakti awakens you to the direct experience of "I am jiva, and I am Shiva. I am the individual bound consciousness, and I am the Infinite expanse of all-encompassing Consciousness." With the full realization of that you regain the radical freedom to see each moment in a way that you've never seen it before, opening up possibilities for showing your boundless love, creativity, wisdom, and compassion in any situation. This is extraordinarily expansive for one's consciousness, even on an ego level.

Staying Grounded

However, with that expansive view comes the challenge for the ordinary mind to stay grounded. It's like walking up to a scenic overlook that is at the edge of a high cliff with a drop straight down to the ocean waves crashing on the rocks far below. There's not even a guardrail, and looking out into the vastness of the sea and the expanse of the horizon, so enormous you can see the curvature of the earth, may be a dizzying experience even though your feet are literally on the ground. You might feel like you are about to fall into that vast space or even leap into it, but of course you don't! Falling into the infinite spaciousness of Divine Awareness can be overwhelming, even shattering, to the ordinary ego mind. Thus, in the Bhagavad Gita, Arjuna begged Lord Krishna to stop the vision of the Infinitude, which Krishna had granted Arjuna. It was too overwhelming for Arjuna's mind to bear. He had to return to ordinary consciousness and have his ego mind simply fulfill his dharma serving the Divine with all the skill and dedication he had. That's what the ego mind is given to do in order to stay grounded and skillful in its domain, fulfilling one's dharma. It's very grounding to focus on skillfully and lovingly fulfilling your dharma as a son or daughter, spouse, partner or friend, employer or employee. There may be tumultuous times in sadhana when meditative or yoga practices stir too much energy, and it's most grounding to totally focus on fulfilling one's dharmas and stop other types of practices. '

There are often times in the process of Kundalini unfolding when there's a lot of energy that can feel overwhelming and needs to be grounded. Sometimes that's literally grounding, brought to the earth. The muladhara chakra, the root chakra from which Kundalini typically awakens, is associated with the element earth and with the sense of smell. The feel of earth and the smell of earth can be extraordinarily grounding for individuals. I've worked with people who lived in a big city and found it hard to be in a good earthy environment. But simply growing a plant in a pot, or growing flowers, herbs, tomatoes and having some nice, rich earth right there to smell, touch, and feel, helped them tremendously. Even when you buy a bag of potting soil and you open it, there's a luscious earthy smell to it. That alone, for some people, will ground them immediately. Just opening up a bag of earth and smelling it and putting their hands in it changes their Shakti, changes their energy, changes how the energy is moving through their body and grounds it.

Grounding exercises like those done in bioenergetics therapy can be helpful. These might include working on the soles of the feet, strengthening contact with the ground, rubbing the soles of the feet on the ground or floor while bare foot, stomping, running bare foot on the beach or on the grass, doing intense physical work, and mindfully doing household chores. Shifting your attention away from whatever is happening energetically and focusing on acting skillfully and mindfully in the moment is grounding. The old Zen adage of "chop wood, carry water, when hungry eat, when thirsty drink," is grounding advice. You train the mind not to get carried away by unusual sensations, visions, and so forth. You simply focus on doing what is dharmic and necessary in the moment. Let go and let Shakti.

You may discover that Kundalini guides you to ground it in ways that are just what you need. People have told me that they found they had to walk barefoot for a while each day or walk out in the woods, that it was a craving for some period of time, but it had never been there before so they wondered if they were going crazy! No, they needed to ground the energy and were being led to how best to do that for themselves. Walking along the ocean or along a body of water, being outside, and being in the elements are very grounding for Kundalini as well. When you read descriptions of some of the auspicious sites for doing sadhana in the yogic scriptures, the environments that were most auspicious, most conducive, were the forest, near a body of water, near a river, near the ocean, or in the mountains—all grounding, pure environments. Even people in urban areas like New York City have told me they went out and made their way to Central Park and walked through the grass and the woods there because it was a grounding environment. It helped to quiet their energies, and they felt more harmony and stillness within themselves. In sadhana, you become aware of the kinds of elements, activities, and even food that you need to be grounded.

These kinds of experiences and these ways of working with the energy change as we progress and as we gain greater and greater freedom. Often the initial experiences of Kundalini awakening are the most tumultuous times because it's the time when the movement of Shakti is encountering the most areas in the body and the mind that need to be cleared and opened. As time goes by, the process becomes more subtle, more gentle, more expansive, more ecstatic and love-drenched!

There's a simple Buddhist daily practice that also helps to keep the ego mind grounded and aware of its reality. The practice is called the five remembrances and is based on the Buddha's teachings about the ephemeral, ceaselessly changing nature of all forms. The ego clings to a false sense of permanence, a false self, and this practice helps to cut through that as well. The five remembrances are:

1. There is no escaping aging. I too will grow old.
2. There is no escaping physical degeneration. My body will grow weaker.
3. There is no escaping death. I will die.
4. Everything and everyone changes; we must part from all those we love.
5. My deeds are always with me as propensities. Only my karma accompanies me when I die. My karma is the ground on which I stand.

It's very sobering for the mind to contemplate these five remembrances every day. Try it for just two weeks and see what happens. You may want to continue it every day as His Holiness the Dalai Lama has since he was a child. By focusing on one's karma, one's actions, and the consequences they give rise to, the ego mind stays grounded. It remains in a position to be the skillful servant, mindful in the moment.

Viewing the mind and body as vehicles of consciousness provides additional important insights. When you own a car, you go out, drive your car to where you're going, get out of it, and leave it behind. You're not identified with your car (hopefully not!). You know it's a vehicle; it gets you around in this world. It may suffer some dents, it may get dirty, and you have to take care of it—take it to the car wash, perhaps take it in for repairs—but you don't suffer the experience directly of what it is to be the car. You don't get in and become your car, regardless of auto advertising! And if its idle is a little rough, you don't feel really horrible because "boy, I'm idling rough today." No, it's your vehicle, you'll take care of it, you'll get it fixed, you'll get better fuel, you'll make sure it's well maintained, but it's just a vehicle. It's not you.

That kind of detached and expansive awareness informs the mind as we broaden the view of our experience and see more clearly what the containers of our consciousness are that we inhabit—the vehicles of mind and body. Entering that awareness gives us the freedom to step back and look at these forms that we've created, the forms of mind and body as vehicles of consciousness. This empowers us to act on them by seeing them clearly, and we can see how they can be transformed. As long as we're identified with something, we're attached to it, we'll defend it, and we'll be blind to things about it. Even on a level of how to work with the mind skillfully, regardless of Kundalini, cultivating the capacity to be detached and aware, able to view the mind and body with compassion from a place of equanimity and kindness, frees one from many of the conditioned responses, the triggers that provoke anger, irritability, defensiveness, and unconsciousness.

Some people are so disconnected from their body for a wide variety of reasons that they actually need to be more connected to and more sensitive about their physical vehicle. Hatha yoga practices, qigong, tai chi, bodywork, massage therapy, and other therapeutic techniques can be important components of a person's sadhana.

TRAUMATIC LIFE EXPERIENCES

One of the things I've noticed over the decades of working with people is that individuals who have had a great deal of trauma in their lives, and tragically there are a lot of people who have suffered through many different traumas—child abuse or neglect, violence in the family, terrorist attacks, wars, and so many other things that our human psyches have to live through—may have very challenging experiences with the movement of Shakti Kundalini. They have a lot to clear; there's a lot of bound energy. They've had to wall off a lot in order to even survive the traumas that they've been through. They've had to develop certain kinds of strengths, but at the same time they've had to block certain aspects of experiences that could be overwhelming. This allowed them to make it to where they are now, receiving the grace of Kundalini awakening.

Shakti seeks to set a person completely free, and it can open the doors to experiences that were locked in the body, locked in the muscles, locked in the nervous system, locked in the depths of the unconscious that need to be cleared. That may be very challenging for a person. People need to have the kinds of help and support that will get them through all that. This can involve getting professional help from a transpersonal psychologist or psychotherapist, somebody who has an integrative approach to working with trauma and PTSD, somebody who understands how the body and the mind need to be supported through this process in ways that it really deserves and needs in order to resolve these issues. Many times people need more than a simple practice that comes out of a yogic or meditative tradition. They need to work their way through what that trauma is or what the mind encoded or got locked into because of that trauma. They need the company of somebody who walks with them through that experience and guides them to where they can become free of it. That requires special skills, training, and one-on-one availability that most yoga teachers and meditation teachers don't have.

The yogic and meditative traditions have basically assumed that the person coming to these practices is a relatively healthy, intact, and a spiritually motivated individual. Look at just the yamas and niyamas, and you'll see that even the basic lifestyle of a dedicated practitioner is very demanding. These traditions weren't looking at helping a person through deep trauma from abuse, rape, physical injury, violence, disease, or any of the other ghastly things that our human souls may go through. These experiences require special attention in order for one to skillfully move through them. The ordinary practices alone that come out of a meditative or Kundalini tradition are not going to sufficiently support people who have been through such harrowing experiences. If you've been through any of these types of experiences, then by all means, seek out the kind of help that you need. Individuals who are trained in transpersonal psychology, Jungian psychology, or integrative holistic care are more likely to have both an appreciation of Kundalini processes as well as the professional training for supporting a person through the psychological processes of healing and transformation that are part of the larger process of Kundalini unfolding. Too often I've met people who felt they were failing at their spiritual or yogic practices, but it was the practices or the teachers that were failing to meet their needs for healing and processing what they had been through in life. Compassion for oneself dictates that you seek the best type of support for your needs.

There are times when people in the midst of Kundalini processes are drawn to healers or energy workers in order to try to lower their energy level and ease the disruptions that kriyas may be causing. One has to use discrimination because the energy of the healer or their way of working can actually have the opposite effect. People feeling too much energy running through their system from Kundalini awakening usually don't need more energy. It's rare to find the healer who has the capacity to harmonize that kind of excessive energy and ground it. Use your discrimination, watch what the effects of a treatment are, notice how Shakti responds within you. Just because a person may be a very good healer and able to help many people doesn't mean they are skilled at working with Kundalini or with what's going on with your unique system. You may need something different from what they offer, and that's not disparaging the energy worker or healer.

CHRONIC ILLNESSES

Some people encounter pain or chronic illness as a part of their sadhana even if they aren't blessed by awakened Kundalini, or it may be part of their experience of Kundalini unfolding. It's not caused by Kundalini, but it is something that needs special attention to work through in Kundalini sadhana. There was a time when Kundalini awakening and the practices that engendered it were very tightly held secrets. Primarily the only people experiencing them were advanced adepts, people who had been practicing various forms of yoga practices or Buddhist practices for many, many years, if not lifetimes. But we are in an age now when many people are having spontaneous experiences of Kundalini, and they're not coming to that experience with the perfectly healthy yogic body, with a clear and disciplined mind, and living the pure lifestyle created by adherence to the yamas and niyamas.

Kundalini works with anybody and everybody exactly where they are from that moment of awakening onward. Someone may experience Kundalini awakening in the midst of profound illness and Shakti works with that. We have to recognize that we may need people on our sadhana support team who are professionals in various medical fields, who may not have an understanding of yoga, meditation, Shakti, and the like. When we see a medical professional, we want to give them all of our medical history and all the symptoms we're experiencing so they can determine whether the symptoms have a physical or medical basis. It may only confuse the picture if we launch into a discourse on Kundalini, the chakras, and nadis! Just asking a professional if they have any familiarity with yoga, meditation, and their effects on the body and mind can give you a sense of their interest and background. They don't necessarily have to know about these things to be of help, but their answer may give you a sense of what will be beneficial for you to discuss about yoga processes or Kundalini with them.

For individuals who are challenged by diseases or chronic illnesses, while at the same time going through Kundalini unfolding, Kundalini's empowerment can give people the experience of being supported from within by Shakti and given access to Witness Consciousness that allows them to observe the body and mind with greater detachment and patience. When I was with Swami Muktananda at his ashrams in the United States and India, I was given the seva to help run a clinic and work with individuals who were going through various challenges, both health challenges as well as mental and emotional challenges. There were individuals with many different kinds of disorders, some quite severe, and in need of ongoing medical treatment and medications. They had Kundalini awakening and were going through that along with the challenges of whatever their medical condition was. The practices, mantra, and the grace of Kundalini supported them through what can be a lifelong process.

Some people would think, "Maybe I shouldn't be on medication; Shakti should just take care of it," and Baba would say something like, "What do you think the medication is? Who do you think created the medication? It's Shakti that takes that form so that you can do sadhana and become free." He would tell people, "You don't go off your medication. You take your medication when needed, and you do your sadhana." When it comes to getting medical treatment, use your discrimination, do what supports you the best. I've worked with people on medications or in treatment for a wide range of illnesses, both mental and physical, and Kundalini-empowered practices can work congruently with what they need medically.

INVOKING SHAKTI'S HEALING PRESENCE

One way of helping our body and mind cope with challenging experiences is remembering Kundalini Shakti as the Great Mother, the one who gives her devotees all the support and care they need, whose nature is loving, kind, and healing. Invoke her presence through prayer and contemplation, perhaps using images of the Divine Feminine that resonate for you, along with the unlimited power of mantra—her sound form. There may be times when one needs to really immerse the mind in a practice of invoking Her over and over again, moment by moment. That can be done through the practice of merging the mind in one of the great mantras that invoke her presence as the Great Mother. Om Kali Ma is a maha mantra, a great mantra that invokes Ma Kali, who has the power to cut through all obstacles. She protects her devoted followers from anything that may arise. Repeat Om Kali Ma, Om Kali Ma. Whether you are repeating that silently or out loud, at the same time envision the presence of the Divine that comes to your mind, to your heart, and keep coming back to that. Be patient, the Divine moves from the domain of the eternal, where time, as our ego mind experiences it, does not exist.

What is that loving or caring presence? What is that presence of a protector, or of a nurturer, or one who wards off danger? That one may take different forms at different times, even while you keep coming back to the mantra Om Kali Ma, Om Kali Ma, as quickly or slowly, loudly or gently as you need to in the moment. The forms appear to ease the mind and give it a grace-bestowing form to relate to. The essential power is formless. It can take the form of a sage or saint, a god or goddess, an animal, an angel, or pure light.

One can use a great mantra from the Buddhist tradition such as Om Tare Tum Soha, an invocation of Red Tara, the powerful form of Buddha's boundless compassion that brings to the seeker anything needed to ease the way forward, to remove obstacles and support the seeker. Om Tare Tum Soha, Om Tare Tum Soha, take refuge in Tara, take refuge in Om Tare Tum Soha. These mantras are ways that we can invoke that protective, nurturing presence of the Infinite.

In the Christian tradition there's what could be considered a Latin mantra: Sancta Maria Mater Dei. It invokes Mother Mary, mother of God. One can invoke her presence, bring her to heart, and take refuge in her—Sancta Maria Mater Dei, ease the burdens of the mind and body. In that way countless devotees of Christ have taken refuge in the Holy Mother and found her supportive presence carries them through the most difficult and challenging times. Sancta Maria Mater Dei as a mantra can be repeated over and over again, giving the mind a safe refuge to rest in.

TRANSCEND AND INCLUDE

By stepping back from mind and body, viewing them as vehicles, we begin transcending and including them in our consciousness in a much broader way. Too often the blind spots we have about our personality, our mind, our body, and our ways of acting and interacting prevent us from being as effective as we could be in supporting the changes that Kundalini is creating. By detaching from the mind and body, viewing them from a transcendent perspective that isn't identified with them and doesn't need to deny their afflictions or defend their shortcomings, you see clearly what needs to be transformed by self-effort as well as by grace. You are empowered to transform the body-mind vehicle, the container in which your consciousness moves through your life. If it doesn't steer or drive or run the way it should, you can change that. Many times people are astonished to have the experience spontaneously as Kundalini awakens that detached awareness for them. We can also cultivate an expansive view, sustaining it for longer and longer periods of time.

When we've separated awareness to some degree from the mind-body complex, differentiating an observing Witness, we can then act on the mind-body complex with greater ease and skill. In this expansive process engendered by Kundalini, your innate intelligence is unfolding, and you can view the mind and body as vehicles of consciousness. Because you're no longer so identified with the mind-body, you have much greater freedom to examine it, to be fully conscious of its miraculous workings as well as its shortcomings, and to re-create it. Because we have the power to fully sense and feel what this vehicle experiences, we can also be fully conscious of and sensitive to how this wondrous mind-body vehicle allows us to know the world and our interactions with others. This is much more fun than just getting in a car and driving!

Meditation empowered by Kundalini gives us the experience of completely letting go of mind-body identification to know the Infinite, as well as giving us the experience of what it is to re-inhabit, by choice, the vehicles and containers (mind-body, roles, relationships, etc.) we've created to experience the life we are in, without being trapped by sole identification with them.

You can know yourself at the profound level where you are free of all conditioning. Kundalini and the consciousness/meditative disciplines invite everyone to step back and look at these containers, the ego identities, and know that they can be transcended and transformed to serve the highest with love and compassion. For some people, the initial realization of how fluid and self-constructed reality is can be quite unsettling. The ego mind needs to stay grounded in fulfilling its responsibilities, the dharma of our life, even while these larger domains of consciousness open before us.

Remember from the discussion of the psychology of yoga that the ego mind is described as the power of self-appropriation. It appropriates things to itself through the process of identification. It takes on the body, roles, relationships, feelings, the states of waking, dream, and deep sleep, and so on. Those are all the containers that Kundalini both transforms and frees consciousness from so you can know who you are beyond the confines of those containers. By transforming the containers, they become better able to serve your highest nature and participate in manifesting the boundless love, compassion, and wisdom that are your very nature. In this way, the vehicles of mind and body are embraced, transformed, and included as integral to realizing the great purposes of a human birth.

PRAYER

Prayer is a very powerful beda upaya practice. For many people, it connects them with the living presence of the Divine, both within themselves and in the universe, and reorients the ego mind when dealing with challenges. Through surrendered prayer, we receive the infusion of grace we need to persevere, to overcome difficulties, or to gain the wisdom we need from a situation. Prayer opens us to the unimaginable creative impulses and solutions that the grace-bestowing power of the Divine, Shakti Kundalini, can manifest in our lives. Surrendered prayer has as its basis the attitude of "thy will be done" instead of the ego mind's agenda of what it wants to happen. It's another practice that moves the ego mind toward letting go, and many people find it especially helpful during challenging periods of sadhana. Kundalini is a living presence. She is the life of our life. She invites you to relate to Her, to bring to Her your love and devotion, your pain and your longing, frustration and anger, your need for strength and guidance, for patience and compassion. People discover the best way to invoke her loving presence for themselves.

Early on in my sadhana, I didn't relate to prayer. It wasn't until I was in the hospital at age twenty-four and it looked like I might be dying that I genuinely reached out/in to the Divine through prayer. The response was overwhelming with my Lady of Light and Baba appearing in a vision. For me, it is a practice of love and compassion, of entering into a deeply loving awareness of my conventional self's intimate connection with the Divine, and resting in that space of near union, without merger, that allows for the experience of the nectar of Divine love to suffuse the soul. In that space, the ones I'm praying for are with me in my heart. I may see their faces, and the love for them arises. I simply pray that the light and grace of the Divine illumines their way, heals their wounds, and gives them all the wisdom, strength, and support they need to move forward with their soul's journey. Out of the stillness of that sacred space, thoughts and feelings may arise from the ordinary mind that wishes for a particular outcome. They are viewed with compassion and understanding as they pass by and dissolve into stillness once again.

It's easiest for me to pray for others. My Buddhist teachers taught me to pray that whatever pain or suffering this mind and body might be going through, may it in some way help to reduce the suffering of others. I don't know that it ever will, but one thing is clear, when my awareness shifts to the loving compassion that arises for others and their suffering, my pain always diminishes. Pain of any kind can throw the ego mind into a terribly contracted state as it collapses into its pain and losses. Shifting attention to caring for others and recognizing their suffering helps the mind come back to a more expanded state, with greater access to generosity, wisdom, patience, and compassion.

There are many wonderful written works on prayers of invocation, prayers of adoration, prayers of celebration, prayers of petition, prayers of supplication, and centering prayers available to those interested in this way of the heart. Following is a prayer practice that you might find helpful.

PRAYER PRACTICE

Allow your awareness to settle as you would for going into meditation. It may be helpful to have an altar where you light a candle and have pictures or statues or representations of what you love and deeply revere. Love embraces you, those you care for, and the Divine Presence. As you close your eyes and allow your attention to rest inside, bring your awareness to your heart, the center of love, the center of your being. Within the heart there is a living flame like that of a candle that is the living flame of Love, the living presence of the Divine within you. You can draw near to that flame and feel its gentle warmth and loving presence. In your heart are also the ones who care for you, the ones you love, the ones you've brought into the presence of the Divine to receive the light and grace of that One. You don't have to do anything. Just be present there with those whom you are bringing into this prayerful sacred place. The Divine knows what to do. The light, warmth, and love of the Divine will envelop and permeate their souls, helping them in ways seen and unseen. There may be times when the flame of Love burns brighter and taller; there may be times when the gracious flames of the Divine even touch you and those you are praying for, as you sit in awe and wonder, love, and reverence. Linger as long as you like in communion with the Divine. When you are ready to leave, offer a prayer of gratitude thanking the One for its grace, bow, and take your leave. Return as often as you like. The living flame of Love is always there for you.

16

Shedding Light on the Shadow

Carl Jung, the great Swiss psychiatrist, talked about *the shadow* as the dark side of ourselves, the split-off and disowned aspects of ourselves that we are unconscious of because they reside in the shadows of unawareness. The process of spiritual growth and integration—what he called the *individuation process*—included being able to shed light on one's shadow, illuminating the shadow in order to free energy that's bound up in it. The dark side isn't all negative; it's dark in that it is unknown. There are also positive aspects, hidden talents, and unrealized potentials in the shadow that can be brought into the light to blossom. These may be talents and abilities that weren't recognized or nurtured as we were growing up and receded into the shadow through neglect. In Kundalini sadhana, we may be directed by Shakti into the shadow to free unconscious parts of ourselves, to see both negative and positive aspects of the ego mind, and free whatever energy is bound up in them. There are hidden aspects of our self that are radiant and full of extraordinary creativity that are also waiting in the shadow for freedom and illumination.

One of the positive archetypes whose potentials are often lost in that shadow is the divine child, our inner source of creativity, wonder, and direct connection to the Divine, the transcendent one. Our wonderment is a way of being present and connected with the world, and the experience of wonder shares similarities with the Zen notion of "beginner's mind." Think of a child's living sense of wonder; it embodies delight, freedom, spontaneity, and effortless presence because there's an openness to what's right in front of them. Awakened Kundalini reconnects us to what is lost in the shadow—including the wonder and creativity within. It illumines every aspect of who we are.

The hidden elements of our psyche are unknown to ourselves, but they're often not in darkness to anyone else! Other people see our shadow sides and can help illumine them for us. The tricky part is that our ego mind is often deeply invested in not seeing it. Shadow is often denial; shadow develops through an active process of denying a part of us that exists. It doesn't wind up in the shadow by accident; it's there on purpose, driven there by parents, family, teachers, ourselves, and others. People also add to their shadow by unconsciously denying the parts that don't fit in with how they are trying to project themselves in groups and in relationships or how they are trying to project their spirituality. Integrative sadhana demands that we consciously transform and reclaim our shadow energy, adding to the relative freedom of the mind.

One of the ways that we can help to retrieve what's in the shadow is to consciously approach the shadow, bringing the light of awareness into that place. This exercise can be done repeatedly at different times, whenever you're feeling stuck, whenever you're saying, "Hmmm, things are going really well, I wonder what's lurking in the shadow that still needs to be drawn out." This invites the wisdom and power of what is hidden there to come forward and allows you to be there to receive it and to learn from it.

INVITING THE SHADOW INTO THE LIGHT OF AWARENESS

Start by sitting comfortably, closing your eyes and allowing your breath to slow and deepen. Bring your mind to the Witness, and allow the mind to settle into a safe and comfortable space of being detached and aware, relaxed and at ease, protected and secure. Sometimes you might even find that there are particular protectors that you ask to be there with you, or it might be the feeling of being wrapped in a luminous shield of mantra. Imagine you are in a large comfortable room; it's nighttime, perhaps there's fire in the fireplace, and you sit cozy and at ease with your protectors or by yourself. You can see that there are dark shadows in the corners of the room, behind some of the furniture, and there's a dark hallway leading off from the far end of the room. You can sense something or someone in the shadows who would like to come out, but needs some encouragement. You invite them to come into the warm inviting light. Simply watch with patience and compassion as whatever it is chooses to come forward. It may be a person, an animal, a mythic being, or something else. Now you might engage that aspect in a dialogue, asking what message it might have for you or what it would like to show you. Take as much time as you need with this being. What does it need? What does it want? How can it be set free?

When it is time to part, do so with appreciation for it coming forward. If you need to return to it to learn more, set a time to do that. The shadow wants to be related to, to be freed, to release its power so that the whole psyche has more energy. You might want to journal about your experiences of the shadow sides of yourself, what you've discovered, how these parts can be freed and integrated.

SHADOW WORK: EXPANDING FREEDOM FROM SUFFERING

Our psyche has many parts that may need transformation, freedom, redemption, or reclamation. The shadow is the most hidden aspect of those parts. We also have wounded parts, creative parts, wise parts, childish parts, perfectionist parts, rebellious parts, and on and on. Some are in deeper shadow than others. Some we have partial awareness of, even if it is after they seize our mind-body vehicle and run it off the road! Shadow work needs to be done to fully integrate our spiritual development and transform these hidden aspects of the ego mind that create suffering for ourselves and for others. During Witness meditations and mindfulness meditations, we often see the mental patterns that make up these parts. The practices empower us to transcend, transform, subsume, and integrate these parts into a more functional whole. By accessing states of expanded awareness that can look at the mind in its totality, seeing the light and dark aspects from a perspective of compassion, wisdom, and love, we can see the afflicted mind states that are especially apparent in our shadow and others as well. We can cultivate the patience and compassion needed to contain and transmute the shadow. Kundalini often dissolves our identification with many of these parts quite effortlessly and releases the energy bound in them. We can work in alignment with Kundalini's intention to make us awake, aware, and free of our shadow.

Often we project our shadow onto others. One quick way to start seeing your shadow is to look at people whom you have an immediate negative reaction to, often before you know them at all. Look at your reaction, and examine what it is about them that is annoying, irritating, revolting, and so forth. Now look at who you know who has those qualities, especially if the qualities are in close family members, parents, brothers or sisters, aunts or uncles, or if those qualities can be seen in close friends, teachers, or someone else you spent a lot of time with, or someone who may have had power over you. Lastly, look for those qualities inside yourself. When do you say to yourself, "I hate it when I ____." That's an indicator of shadow, of something rejected that's looking to get free. Any energy we have tied up in holding those qualities in the unconscious, holding them back from being acted out, is energy that is tied up and unavailable. Those shadow qualities need to be worked through to be set free, not freely acted out, but set free so that there's nothing there that has to be forced below the surface. Sometimes that is best done with a psychologist or therapist.

Shadow work frequently happens spontaneously in the process of Kundalini unfolding, and there will be many times as one meditates when those shadow aspects come up to reveal themselves. They're suddenly simply present in your awareness. Many years ago when I was new to the path of Kundalini and going through a lot of very dramatic kinds of activity, movements of mind, movements of body, visions, and the like, I was sitting in meditation and suddenly what came up was something quite mundane and shadow-related.

Two years prior, I had borrowed money from my employer to buy a car from her. What came up was that I had missed a payment. We had arranged monthly payments, and I was away on vacation and had missed a payment, and I had failed to recognize it. She didn't catch it either. But somehow in that moment, my shadow had skipped the payment and also missed catching it. In the mystical Sufi tradition, the shadow side is called the *nafs*. The shadow sides of us can be very subtle, as well as large and obvious to others. They can cause huge crash-and-burn events or create little trip-ups or little karmas of indebtedness.

After meditation when this came to mind, I went to my employer, Dr. Renee Nell, who was also a mentor of mine. She was an elder Jungian analyst and had trained with Carl Jung and M. Esther Harding, another great Jungian analyst. I told her what had happened in meditation that day and she laughed and got a kick out of it and said, "Ah, the shadow side!" And I said, "Yes, and thank goodness for the side of us that illumines it!" The power of Consciousness, Kundalini Shakti is always shedding light on our shadow. Of course, I paid her my missing payment with interest; I didn't want any karmic indebtedness!

When we realize that some part of the shadow has done something negative, whether that realization comes in meditation or through an insight or someone telling us, then we have to make amends. It's like in twelve-step programs, when you see something that you've done wrong. You don't just say, "Oh, ok, I see it now." You make amends as best the ego mind can. You act in a way to heal that situation, to change it. You stay present and recognize what needs to be done internally as well as externally. You also commit to remaining conscious and not doing it again.

It's significant that in an ancient hymn to Kundalini Shakti, the Kundalini Stavaha, it says that the person who gains full realization through Kundalini is the one who wants to become free and is aware of their faults and shortcomings.[1] It's not enough to just want true freedom, we also have to be aware of what our ego mind's faults are, what the shortcomings are of our conventional self. We have to do that shadow work, we have to illumine all aspects of our psyche and set them free. We have to have unimpeded clarity of vision.

When people transcend to escape—and they do this quite frequently—they slow their progress and create more karmas to work through. This doesn't transform and include the domains where a person is stuck and seeks escape through transcendence. When a person comes back from the transcendent experience, all they're doing is bringing more power into these untransformed aspects of their mind. The ego mind uses the transcendent experience to deny the presence of the untransformed shadow aspect. People then act out their bondage with more energy. It's incumbent upon us as seekers, as devotees of Kundalini Shakti, as devotees of whatever our own path may be, to go into the shadow realms of our own psyches and transform them. Radical freedom is all-inclusive.

Part of that process is asking for and being open to candid feedback from others. Too often on a spiritual path, people become spiritualized, and that too is a shadow aspect of the ego mind that co-opts and tries to own that it's becoming transcendent; it's owning its attainment as if it's above and beyond these negative patterns that it once had. With that shadow dynamic, the ego mind has deluded itself into thinking it has left them behind, and so it doesn't even want to hear the feedback that other people are giving it. We have to be open to feedback; we have to invite feedback so that we can see the shadow sides of ourselves. This is part of what a teacher provides. It's not enough to have a statue on our puja or the picture of a dead master or saint. That makes it too easy for the ego mind to hide its shadow sides. It's risky for the ego mind to relate to a living teacher. A teacher with integrity will give feedback in a compassionate way. There are so many beliefs about how a student should relate to a teacher that block feedback from being a two-way communication. Yet rules of absolute surrender and respect were only meant to apply to true selfless, enlightened masters. Many teachers need feedback as much as or more so than some students.

We really are dependent on the feedback of others, of honest teachers, mentors, our sangha, and those whom we love and trust, but often the universe is giving us feedback if we're willing to listen, if we're not invested in denial. How somebody treats us waiting in line, how somebody treats us when we get to the checkout counter in a store, and how we treat that person, how we react is feedback. Daily life gives us feedback, and becoming aware of it is part of the process of unfolding Kundalini, of expanding consciousness. It isn't just going into blissful states, kriyas, visions, and ecstatic union with Shiva and Shakti dancing in the sahasrara! Though that is very enjoyable, it's going down into the mud, it's going down into the darkness, because She also revels in clearing that up.

EGO SELF-CHERISHING

One of the aspects of the ego mind that needs transforming, though it doesn't often consider it (thus it can be buried in shadow), is that it is always involved with itself. There's a self-cherishing dimension to the ego mind—and this aspect of the ego definitely needs to be brought to light. It's always engaged with its thoughts, its feelings, or its view of itself or others' view of it with a kind of fascination that outside of sadhana would just be considered normal. There's an inherent narcissism to the ego mind that's its conditioned nature, that's part of its structure, but it's also part of what the unfolding of Kundalini and the deepening of spiritual practice always confronts and transforms. It's an aspect of the ego mind that we're not stuck with; it's an aspect of the ego mind that we can change so that it becomes the best servant of our own highest nature. Kundalini-empowered practices of meditation, mantra, and contemplation cut the root of ego's self-cherishing. Seva is an important practice for transforming the ego mind and integrating the shift away from self-centeredness into everyday life.

We also have to watch the ego mind's spiritual cravings, its cherished experiences that it wants repeated or augmented, because these bind it as well. As transpersonal experiences unfold, they give the ego mind another whole menu that it begins to look at and then says to itself, "Oh, I can have experiences of Shiva and Shakti, and I can have experiences of Buddha and *dakinis* (energetic beings in female form)!" It begins to develop its shopping list of spiritual experiences that it would like to have, or ones that it's had and it's so attached to that it wants to have them again. It's important to keep stepping back and letting go, stepping back and letting go. That's why the sadhana of Kundalini is really the sadhana of surrender, allowing whatever is unfolding in the moment to be received as a gift of Kundalini Shakti and that's it. You may sit for an hour a day, day after day, for year after year, with no "experiences" at all, because that's the gift, being free from needing or craving any experience. Just being able to watch with detached dispassion the ordinary play of the mind is a profound and useful gift of freedom. At other times there may be numinous revelations and they'll come and go. Having the detached dispassion to view the river of Consciousness and all that floats by with equanimity is one of the gifts of awakening. That is also what we're cultivating through the practices done daily with dedication and enthusiasm.

FALSE TRANSCENDENCE

The mind's often desperate need for relief from pain, pain born of identification with the limited or afflicted ego mind, can combine with the yearning for transcendence to produce an escapist or false transcendence. Some people call this a spiritual bypass. It is usually unconscious, another aspect of a person's shadow. Too often the quick fix for obtaining relief from pain appears to be gained through various types of false transcendence, including the use of drugs and alcohol to make one numb and unconscious. A person can use meditation and spiritual disciplines to become numb and unconscious while convincing themselves they are deepening their attainment.

There are many people who have fallen into addiction, genuinely seeking something of transcendence, genuinely seeking to get free of the pain their soul feels, the restrictions, and the confinement that the afflicted ego mind imposes, but then the means, the addictive substance, is even more debilitating. It was Carl Jung who in speaking with Bill, the founder of the Alcoholics Anonymous twelve-step program, said that there was a real spiritual component to the struggle against addiction. Jung seeded the idea of turning to a higher power, the transcendent function, the Self.

When anyone's caught in addiction, the ordinary self flounders and can't get free on its own. People need to turn to a higher power as the ego mind surrenders in order to get free. Surrender in this context doesn't mean giving up, but surrendering the illusion of the all-powerful ego, the self that can overcome obstacles on its own, and surrendering all the denial that goes with that, including the denial of its powerlessness. There is a genuine piece to the soul's yearning for transcendence in addictive patterns that needs to be recognized, but directed in ways that are healthy, skillful, and truly bring relief from suffering.

On any path, one needs to be wary of a yearning to get free of pain via transcendence because it can lead one in directions where the transcendence is false, the illusion of freedom is deeply binding, and the prolonged work it will take to cut through that deluded state can take lifetimes.

ADDICTED TO THINKING

Lest anyone think they're free of addiction and far above this affliction that plagues so many people, try stilling your mind. The mind is addicted to thinking and movement. The ordinary mind is addicted to its flow of thought, feelings, sensations, memories, fantasies about the past and future, and on and on. As I mentioned earlier, when the mind is confronted with the absence of sensory stimuli as it is if you're in a sensory deprivation tank, the conditioned mind becomes so disoriented and craves stimulus to such an extent that it actually produces its own hallucinations!

Zen practitioners have told me about what they called Zen hallucinations that occur during long meditation sittings in *sesshins* (retreat programs that go on for several days). Whole dramas play out before the mind's eye even as they sit motionless staring at the floor in front of them. The ordinary mind, the ego mind, fights the extinguishing of all thought like one fighting to death to stay alive. Indeed, this is what it is doing; so don't be surprised by its tenacity. The ego mind's reality is: "I think, thereby I am." It fears it will die if all movement, all thought ceases. However, you are not your mind. You have a mind, but you're not your mind. Knowing that fully and completely is part of what it means to repossess your radical freedom. The you that already possesses radical freedom is not the you that you've thought yourself to be! We treat the mind with compassion and reassure it that it will continue to exist and thrive even after silence reigns supreme.

Meditation reveals that absolute silence is our womb, our tomb, our refuge, our home.

THE SHADOW SIDE OF GROUPS

Transcendence often means transcending the confines of the ego mind, but it might be an ego mind that's wounded; it might be an ego mind that is restricted because of extreme pains that it has suffered, whether it's through child abuse, trauma, substance abuse and addiction, PTSD, or any number of different circumstances. Often individuals suffering these pains try to seek transcendence and relief in ways that are not empowering. One of the typical forms for this is what happens when people become involved in groups where they surrender their ego mind, in a sense, to the group mind, and it feels more free. It feels more expansive because they're now identifying with the group—this is the root of the dark side of cults, because it often attracts people who are wounded and are seeking to get free of a wounded, restricted self, but they're doing it by getting caught in a group mind that may be equally afflicted or worse. Yet, for the individual, it feels like by merging in the group and becoming empowered by the group and its leader that there's some expansion—even though it is unhealthy, deluded expansion. Every individual is seeking freedom from suffering and the fullness of joy and love. Becoming awake and empowered by Kundalini is the means to do it that brings true freedom and lasting joy.

Some people create false transcendence of the afflicted ego mind through relationships. They feel restricted in themselves, but when they get into a relationship and merge with the other, they feel whole and complete. They become profoundly dependent on that person because the other person is making up for things that they're lacking. There are many ways that co-dependence forms such relationships. It's another way that people try to seek relief through

235

transcendence, but it's not the transcendence that comes from actually contacting our true nature and integrating the power and the strength that come from it. Transcending a wounded self through relationships, merging with partners, teachers or groups, simply keeps the bondage in place.

Another dynamic that happens in the soul's search for transcendence and freedom is the ego mind projecting its nature onto what it thinks freedom is going to be. When the ego mind thinks of freedom, it thinks of getting more and more of what it desires, craves, and has pursued for lifetimes. For some this includes power and fame, which further drives the false guru delusion. Fulfilling the ego's wish list is not the radical freedom that Kundalini will bestow. Your highest nature is seeking the freedom to manifest your true and highest Self with all the boundless compassion, patience, kindness, wisdom, and love that go with that. Until that is fully realized, dharma, the yamas and niyamas, ethical disciplines and practices, dedication to selflessness, seva, compassion, and generosity help to keep the ego mind's deep-rooted self-serving patterns in check.

PSEUDO-ENLIGHTENMENT

A friend and I were out hiking and climbing early one morning. After some hours, we made it to a summit that was open and we were above the clouds. As we rested there for a bit, feeling pretty good about having made it to the top, the sun dissipated the clouds in the distance, and suddenly, we could see that we had only made it to the top of one of the foothills of the mountains we were heading for! Pseudo-enlightenment is like that. Only with pseudo-enlightenment, the shadow side of the ego that wants to appropriate this state to itself, along with whatever goodies it believes go with it, will aggressively deny that there is anything beyond where it is! It defends its delusion and tries to project what it conceives enlightenment to look like. The posturing can be a caricature of the true state of one who has gone beyond, but with all the props that are available, clothes, turbans, robes, collars, and so forth, the afflicted individual can walk the stage of life and gather a following. This is *kali yuga*—it is the age of the shadow, the age of darkness, and a seeker has to bring their own light of discrimination and learning to every moment.

Kundalini graces people with extraordinary experiences, opening expansive vistas that the ordinary mind never imagined existed. The danger is that the ego mind latches onto such experiences, identifies with them, and even fashions a whole new enlightened personality to match its imagined enlightened state. This is a powerful delusion. Without a mentor and a sangha who pop such bubbles of self-inflation, a person can remain trapped in that hall of mirrors for a long time, perhaps tragically drawing in others who also lack the discrimination to see what has happened. Cults form in this way. This delusion has elements of personal shadow as well as the collective shadow of groups that become invested in the "enlightened" stature of their leader and deny all evidence to the contrary that the guru is really in such a lofty state. It can be very difficult for an individual to resist the group-think of a deluded sangha and its leader. No religious or spiritual tradition is immune to this.

The individual caught in pseudo-enlightenment is often so deluded they have no idea they are bound in this way. It is one of the most difficult afflicted ego states to cut through. The poet-saint Kabir suggested that if you find someone claiming to be enlightened, hang them by their feet off a cliff for a few hours and see what state they are in! If they maintain their equanimity maybe you have a real one!

Once I met a Rinpoche, a Tibetan Buddhist master, who had been imprisoned in a Chinese gulag for nearly twenty years. During that time, he was repeatedly beaten, tortured nearly to death on more than one occasion, and lived without any hope of ever regaining his physical freedom. Yet, his one fear during that horrific ordeal was that he might lose his compassion and patience for his torturers and the abusive prison guards. His commitment to Buddhist practice and dharma was absolute. In the gulag he was freer than his Chinese captors. This Rinpoche was one of the kindest, purest, most sublime and humble beings I have ever had the privilege of meeting, all too briefly. He had no malice, no anger, no hatred toward the Chinese for all the untold suffering they have inflicted on him and millions of Tibetans and others. He is a living example of true freedom, true attainment. We are blessed to have living examples of what it is to embody this state. He doesn't have throngs of devotees. He doesn't hold huge public programs. He seeks no fame. He simply lives the practices and precepts of his tradition.

THE SHADOW IN OTHERS

In sadhana we cultivate ways of skillfully working with our own shadow, which empower us to deal with other peoples' dark and afflicted sides as well. The same lessons that come out of mindfulness and Witness Consciousness practices apply. We cultivate the capacity to simultaneously see their divine nature, their Buddha nature, as well as seeing clearly the shrouds of ignorance and fear that create the afflicted states that give birth to the shadow. For this reason, Sage Patanjali recommends that as a yogic practice, you view the wicked with dispassion, with the detached awareness that allows you to see clearly, act skillfully, and prevents you from identifying with being in conflict with or the owner of the afflicted person's projections. That empowers you to remain free, remain clear of conditioned reactivity, and free to respond appropriately, wisely, compassionately, patiently from your true center. Because you've been practicing the same approach internally for dealing with your own shadow, you've expanded your capacity for dealing with the appearance of others in the conventionally agreed upon illusion of an outside world. We really are always and only dealing with ourselves.

THE LIGHT IN THE DARK

The light of Kundalini's transformative fire illumines the dark recesses of our unconscious where gold and jewels of hidden talents and capabilities seem to leap into the present, reveling in the light. People suddenly find themselves inspired to write, draw, sculpt, sing, dance, learn a musical instrument, knit, sew, weave, make jewelry, or bring fresh creativity and ingenuity to their work. Shakti is the creative force of the universe. As the mind and body merge more and more with her flow, that creativity becomes more and more visible in your life. This is her gift. Her generosity knows no bounds. I remember Baba Muktananda saying that Shakti makes a plumber a better plumber, a lawyer a better lawyer, a father a better father, a mother a better mother.

Shakti's creativity and inspiration can infuse any and every aspect of life with grace. The hidden talents and capabilities emerge as the fruit of all the grace and self-effort that has cleared the karmic and psychological muck that buried them. They point toward the grand prize of Self-knowledge, Buddhamind, filled with loving ecstasy that suffuses the instrument of mind-body, making every moment inspired, every action pregnant with revelation. Follow Kundalini's lead with the help of one of her servants. She promises you the radical freedom to know the Infinite at all times and to joyfully serve the One with every breath. This is your birthright. She is within you as you to guarantee that you can attain all that is possible. The gate to the domain of the Infinite opens to her command. Grasp her hand, the sacred mantra, and let Her take you beyond all forms, beyond emptiness, beyond the beyond! Expressed in the mantra of the Heart Sutra:

> Gaté, gaté, paragaté, parasamgaté, bodhi swaha!
> Gone, gone, gone beyond, completely beyond, fully awake, so be it!

May every moment be a meditation and every meditation a revelation!

The Threads, the Cloth, and the Weaver

.

Before awakening, we're barely aware of the fabric of our existence, woven moment by moment by the strands of thought and attention which are snagged on thorns of conditioned ignorance, creating repeating patterns of ephemeral pleasure and pain. Waking up and disciplining the mind with the practices, which work to clear and stabilize our thoughts and attention, prepare the ground for full awakening of Kundalini Shakti. In time we stabilize where our attention goes moment to moment and what it weaves in the process of wandering. Over time we see what happens with attention each moment, and we become aware of how often it wanders off. Where do I want it to be right now? Did it drift off, how do I get it back? How do I keep it focused on the mantra, on the Witness, on cultivating selflessness in the moment? How do I keep it energized, potent, and clear? These are important questions for anybody pursuing meditative practices. Being skillful in sadhana has to do with marshalling the power of our attention because if our attention is wandering, our energy is leaking away, the creative energy of Consciousness, Shakti. How are you leaking Shakti? What do you need to do to tighten your practices?

The light of awareness that is Kundalini shines on the importance of attention. Attention is central to being able to unfold our path and tread it to the end. The practices make us study our attention and look at where it is going. What are we giving it to? Throughout our school years, we were always being told by teachers, "Pay attention! Pay attention. You're not paying attention!" In that was a message: Pay attention! Invest your attention. Attention is an extraordinarily valuable commodity; you could say it's the most valuable commodity. Without attention nothing flourishes. None of your relationships, your goals for a career, your hopes and dreams, nothing comes into being or is sustained or grows without attention.

We in fact know that even human life requires attention. A newborn can be well fed, warm, and comfortable, but without attention they can die, they can literally die. This tragically happens in orphanages that don't have the resources to give the attention that an infant needs. Life itself depends on attention. Your spiritual practices, the unfolding of your highest nature, depends on your attention given fully and enthusiastically to those practices, to living them in the moment.

You might wonder what is the highest attention? Love, love is the highest attention. What we give our love to flourishes. Through love, our attention flows with ease and grace. Cultivate love, the heart of sadhana. Any practice done without love becomes mere drudgery. Don't let the mind dry up the fountain of love that keeps sadhana juicy and alive.

It doesn't take doing sadhana or meditation long before it becomes very clear that lapses of attention are the gaps in which the ordinary mind reasserts itself, with the unconscious processes of our conditioning, whether it's out of fear, irritability, anger, or being driven by some desire, need, or some power trip that we've got. Whatever it might be, these patterns creep into those gaps of inattentiveness. We have to become more and more skilled at sustaining our attention through a unique vigilance that is free of tension. Awakened Kundalini supports that process internally.

One of the hallmarks of awakened Kundalini is that Shakti is always supporting, in every way possible, you remaining conscious, remaining awake and aware. In Kundalini sadhana, you are not just relying on the ordinary mind to sustain your sadhana practices. With shaktipat comes the awakened energy that is driving sadhana forward from within and sustaining the unfolding of our innate capacities for the highest levels of attention and consciousness, beyond anything even the most vigilant ego mind will ever manifest.

The teacher serves you by helping to keep your attention informed and focused on your sadhana. All the practices and teachings that are given by Kundalini and a wise mentor work with your attention in the moment, engaging it in ways that open doors of awareness you may never have known existed. Some doors only open after they have absorbed the energy of years of loving attention. Some hearts are like that as well. In time wisdom and patience will effortlessly flow through you.

Years ago, while I was in meditation, Shakti said to me, "You know it's *your* consciousness; you can change what you are investing it in. Make your conscious attention an offering to God; continually offer your consciousness to God through prayer, meditation, and service, and in time you will see God as everyone, everything, everywhere."

It's all about attention, moment by moment, paying attention, investing your attention and seeing that you can control it and offer it in service to the Divine. Kundalini empowers you to gather all the strands of attention that leak your energy, diminishing the effectiveness of your practices.

Following Shakti Kundalini means giving Her your full attention. And it needn't be a chore! She's inviting you to know the love and bliss of merging your attention, your consciousness in Her! She's saying, "Follow the loving bliss, it will take you beyond suffering! Follow the loving bliss, it is my scent! Follow the loving bliss, it will take you home now!"

She is here, present in the fabric of our lives. Pick up any thread, and you take hold of the whole divine cloth. Pick up any strand, and you take hold of Her. Then She'll show you that it is only Her picking up herself. We don't add tantric practices to life. Tantra is woven in; it's already part of the cloth. Awakening is seeing what is already here and marveling at it, delighting in what it makes apparent, the Infinite permeating your mind, body, and all the world. Shakti opens our eyes to the wonder and splendor of each moment.

As a child, I remember watching a woman combing sheep wool. The little fibers were short and weak. I could easily pull them apart and break them. But the woman would gather them together and spin it into thread. Then she would take several strands of the thread and twist them together into yarn. It was so strong that I couldn't break the piece she handed to me. In this Divine world, there are threads from every tradition and religion in Her cloth, threads of every living creature and every kind of experience, threads of water, earth, fire, and air. She created them all and wove this marvelous cloth from her own being, of which we too are threads. We can merge in her boundless delight of creation! She invites us to know that She is us! She always has been. She's all that is and ever will be. She willingly bears the pain of separation for the unspeakable joy of reunion! Wait no longer. Dissolve in Her embrace!

Emaho!

TARA'S PRAYER

Many pains,
  one cause,
Many clouds,
  one sky,
Many egos,
  one Self,
Many struggles,
  one release,
Many shadows,
  one Light,
Many bonds,
  one freedom,
Many cloths,
  one weaver,
Many ages,
  one eternity,
Many passions,
  one Love,
Many sufferers,
  one cry for compassion,
  patience and Love.
O Beloved Tara,
  answering the cry,
  let us serve 'til
  all are free.

KALIDAS[1]

Notes

SHREE KUNDALINI INVOCATION

1. The Kundalini Stavaha comes from the ancient Rudrayamala Tantra.
   I learned to chant the Kundalini Stavaha in Sanskrit from Swami
   Muktananda in the late 1970s. Christopher Wallis provides an excellent
   online translation of it.

INTRODUCTION: KUNDALINI'S QUEST: THE FULL EMBRACE OF LIFE

1. Joseph Campbell, *The Hero With A Thousand Faces* (Princeton: Princeton
   University Press, 1973), 3.

2. Ibid., 11.

3. Stephen Clissold, trans., *Wisdom of the Spanish Mystics* (New York:
   Directions Publishing Corp., 1977), 32.

4. Non-dual schools of philosophy hold that there is no separation, no duality,
   between creation and Creator, between the transcendent and the immanent.
   There is only one all-encompassing Self or God or Consciousness taking on all
   limited forms of creation while remaining transcendent and infinite as well.

5. V. K. Subramaniam, trans., *Saundaryalahari of Sankaracarya* (Delhi, India:
   Motilal Banarsidass, 1980).

6. M. P. Pandit, trans., *Kularnava Tantra* (Madras, India: Ganesh & Co., 1973).

7. Lawrence Edwards, "Psychological Change and Spiritual Growth Through the Practice of Siddha Yoga" (PhD dissertation, Temple University, 1987).

8. Carl Jung, *Psychological Commentary on Kundalini Yoga, Lectures 1 & 2, 1932* (New York: Spring Publications, 1975), 18.

9. Lawrence Edwards et al., *Kundalini Rising: Exploring the Energy of Awakening*, ed. Tami Simon (Boulder: Sounds True, 2009).

1. KUNDALINI AND THE GREAT GODDESS

1. V. K. Subramanian, trans., *Saundaryalahari* (Delhi, India: Motilal Banarsidass,1980), 1.

2. Lawrence Edwards, *Kali's Bazaar Penned by Kalidas* (Atlanta, Muse House Press, 2012), 49.

2. THE UNIVERSE WITHIN

1. Aldous Huxley, *The Perennial Philosophy* (New York: Harper Colophon, 1970), 11.

3. ENCOUNTERING KUNDALINI: THROUGH THE HEART, BEYOND THE MIND

1. Lex Hixon, *Mother of the Universe* (Wheaton, IL: The Theosophical Publishing House, 1994), 53.

4. MAPS OF KUNDALINI'S DOMAIN

1. Robert Bly, trans., *The Kabir Book* (Boston: The Seventies Press, 1977), 29.

7. YOGA PSYCHOLOGY AND WESTERN PSYCHOLOGY

1. See Thomas Kuhn, *The Structure of Scientific Revolutions* (Chicago University of Chicago Press, 1962) and Roger Walsh, "The Consciousness Disciplines and the Behavioral Sciences: Questions of Comparison and Assessment," *American Journal of Psychiatry,* 137 (1980), 663–73. Much of this discussion of the clash between traditional Western psychology and the Eastern or consciousness disciplines is derived from Walsh's article.

2. See Walsh, "The Consciousness Disciplines and the Behavioral Sciences: Questions of Comparison and Assessment," and Ken Wilber, *Eye to Eye: The Quest for the New Paradigm* (Garden City, NY: Anchor Press/Doubleday, 1983).

3. See Charles Tart, ed., "Some Assumptions of Orthodox, Western Psychology," *Transpersonal Psychologies* (London: Routledge & Kegan Paul, 1975).

4. Fritjof Capra, *The Turning Point* (New York: Bantam Books, 1982), 178.

5. Sigmund Freud, *General Psychological Theory* (New York: Simon & Schuster, 1991), 61.

6. S. Radhakrishnan, trans., *The Principal Upanishads* (New York: Humanities Press, 1978), Taittraya Upanishad, II, 6.

7. Stanislav Grof, "East and West: Ancient Wisdom and Modern Science," *The Journal of Transpersonal Psychology*, 15 (1983),14.

8. See Brandt Dayton, ed., *Practical Vedanta: Selected Works of Swami Rama Tirtha* (Honesdale, PA: Himalayan International Institute of Yoga Science and Philosophy, 1978).

9. Jaideva Singh, trans., *Shiva Sutras* (Delhi, India: Motilal Banarsidass, 1979), 130–31.

10. Jaideva Singh, trans., *Spanda-Karikas* (Delhi, India: Motilal Banarsidass, 1980), 167.

11. Charles Tart, "Some Assumptions of Orthodox, Western Psychology."

12. Swami Prabhavananda, *How to Know God: The Yoga Aphorisms of Patanjali* (Hollywood, CA: Vedanta Press, 1969), 16.

13. Stephen Wilson, "Becoming a Yogi: Resocialization and Deconditioning as Conversion Processes," *Sociological Analysis*, 45 (1984), 301–14.

14. Daniel Goleman and Gary Schwarz, "Meditation as an Intervention in Stress Reactivity," *Journal of Counseling and Clinical Psychology*, 44 (1976), 465.

15. S. Radhakrishnan, trans., *The Principal Upanishads*, Brihadaranyaka Upanishad VI, 22.

16. Lawrence Edwards, "Psychological Change and Spiritual Growth Through the Practice of Siddha Yoga," 139–53.

8. FINDING AND FOLLOWING THE TRUTH THROUGH VIVEKA, DISCRIMINATION

1. Lawrence Edwards, *Kali's Bazaar Penned by Kalidas*, 53.

9. CULTIVATING THE FIELD FOR AWAKENING

1. Lawrence Edwards, *Kali's Bazaar Penned by Kalidas*, 159.

2. Sokei-an Sasaki, *Original Nature: Zen Comments on the Sixth Patriarch's Platform Sutra* (Bloomington: iUniverse, 2012), 82.

3. BeliefNet, accessed October 17, 2007, www.beliefnet.com/Quotes/Buddhist/General/H/His-Holiness-The-Dalai-Lama/It-Is-Critical-To-Serve-Others-To-Contribute-Acti.aspx.

4. Lawrence Edwards, *Kali's Bazaar Penned by Kalidas*, 67.

11. MEDITATION: UNFOLDING KUNDALINI'S GRACE

1. Lawrence Edwards, *Kali's Bazaar Penned by Kalidas*, 57.

2. Lawrence Edwards, *Kali's Bazaar Penned by Kalidas*, 73.

3. Eknath Easwaren, trans., *The Dhammapada* (Tomales, California: Nilgiri Press, 2005), 78.

4. Lawrence Edwards et al., *Kundalini Rising: Exploring the Energy of Awakening*, ed. Tami Simon (Boulder: Sounds True, 2009).

12. THE ROLE OF THE TEACHER/GURU IN KUNDALINI SADHANA

1. Jaideva Singh, trans., *Shiva Sutras*, 102.

2. I. K. Taimni, trans., *The Science of Yoga: The Yoga Sutras of Patanjali* (Wheaton, IL: The Theosophical Publishing House, 1975).

3. Jaideva Singh, trans., *Shiva Sutras*, 103.

13. UPAYAS: THE MEANS TO FREEDOM

1. Jaideva Singh, trans., *Shiva Sutras*, 65.

15. CHALLENGES ON THE PATH

1. Paul Simon, "All Around The World Or The Myth Of Fingerprints" on *Graceland*, Warner Brothers, originally released in 1986.

2. "Akkosa Sutta: Insult" (SN 7.2), translated from Pali by Thanissaro Bhikkhu, accessed September 24, 2012, www.accesstoinsight.org/tipitaka/sn/sn07/sn07.002.than.html.

3. Lawrence Edwards, *Kali's Bazaar Penned by Kalidas*, 75.

16. SHEDDING LIGHT ON THE SHADOW

1. Swami Muktananda, *Kundalini Stavaha* (South Fallsburg, NY: SYDA Foundation 1980), 20.

EPILOGUE: THE THREADS, THE CLOTH, AND THE WEAVER

1. Lawrence Edwards, *Kali's Bazaar Penned by Kalidas*, 61.

Bibliography

Anderson, Sherry and Patricia Hopkins. *The Feminine Face of God.* New York: Bantam Books, 1992.

Aranya, Swami H. *Yoga Philosophy of Patanjali.* 3rd ed. Calcutta, India: Calcutta University Press, 1981.

Ashokananda, Swami, trans. *Avadhuta Gita of Dattatreya.* Madras, India: Sri Ramakrishna Math, 1977.

Begley, Sharon. *Train Your Mind: Change Your Brain.* New York: Ballantine Books, 2007.

Bly, Robert, trans. *The Kabir Book.* Boston: The Seventies Press, 1977.

_____. *Iron John: A Book About Men.* New York: Addison-Wesley Publishing Company, Inc., 1990.

Bly, Robert and Jane Hirshfield. *Mirabai: Ecstatic Poems.* Boston: Beacon Press, 2004.

Bohm, David and John Welwood. "Issues in Physics, Psychology and Metaphysics: A Conversation." *The Journal of Transpersonal Psychology,* 12 (1980): 25–36.

Campbell, Joseph. *The Hero With a Thousand Faces.* Princeton: Princeton University Press, 1973.

_____. *Transformations of Myth Through Time.* New York: Harper and Row, 1990.

Campbell, Joseph, Riane Eisler, Marija Gimbutas, and Charles Musès. *In All Her Names: Explorations of the Feminine in Divinity.* San Francisco: Harper, 1991.

Chatterji, J. C. *Kashmir Shaivism.* Chandigarh, India: Galav Publications, 1981.

Clissold, Stephen. *Wisdom of the Spanish Mystics.* New York: New Directions Publishing Corp., 1977.

Corby, James et al. "Psychophysiological Correlates of the Practice of Tantric Yoga Meditation." *Archives of General Psychiatry,* 35 (1978): 571–77.

Cragg, Kenneth. *The Wisdom of the Sufis.* New York: New Directions Publishing Corp., 1976.

Das, Lama Surya. *Awakening the Buddha Within.* New York: Broadway Books, 1997.

Davidson, Richard and Sharon Begley. *The Emotional Life of Your Brain.* New York: Hudson Street Press, 2012.

Dayton, Brandt, ed. *Practical Vedanta, Selected Works of Swami Rama Tirtha.* Honesdale, PA: Himalayan Institute, 1978.

Easwaren, Eknath, trans. *The Dhammapada: The Sayings of the Buddha.* Tomales, CA: Nilgiri Press, 2005.

Edwards, Lawrence. "Psychological Change and Spiritual Growth Through the Practice of Siddha Yoga." PhD diss., Temple University, 1987. University Microfilms International.

_____. *The Soul's Journey: Guidance From The Divine Within.* Lincoln, NE: iUniverse, 2000.

_____. *Kali's Bazaar Penned by Kalidas.* Atlanta: Muse House Press, 2012.

Edwards, Lawrence et al. *Kundalini Rising: Exploring the Energy of Awakening,* edited by Tami Simon. Boulder: Sounds True, 2009.

Eisler, Riane. *The Chalice & The Blade.* San Francisco: Harper, 1988.

Evans-Wentz, W. Y., ed. *Tibet's Great Yogi Milarepa.* New York: Oxford University Press, 1969.

Feldman, Christina and Jack Kornfield, eds. *Stories of the Spirit, Stories of the Heart: Parables of the Spiritual Path from Around the World.* San Francisco: Harper, 1991.

Feuerstein, Georg. *Tantra: The Path of Ecstasy.* Boston: Shambhala, 1998.

_____. *The Yoga Tradition: Its History, Literature, Philosophy and Practice.* Chino Valley, AZ: Hohm Press, 2001.

Frawley, David. *Inner Tantric Yoga: Working with the Universal Shakti.* Twin Lakes, WI: Lotus Press, 2008.

Galland, China. *Longing For Darkness: Tara and the Black Madonna.* New York: Penguin, 2007.

Goleman, Daniel. "Meditation and Consciousness: An Asian Approach to Mental Health." *American Journal of Psychotherapy,* 30 (1976): 41–54.

Goleman, Daniel and Gary E. Schwartz. "Meditation as an Intervention in Stress Reactivity." *Journal of Counseling and Clinical Psychology,* 44 (1976): 456–66.

Grof, Stanislav. "East and West: Ancient Wisdom and Modern Science." *Journal of Transpersonal Psychology,* 15 (1983): 13–36.

Guenther, Herbert. *The Life and Teachings of Naropa.* New York, Oxford University Press, 1971.

Gyatso, Lama Tenzin (H. H. the Dalai Lama). *Essence of the Heart Sutra: The Dalai Lama's Heart Wisdom Teachings.* Translated and edited by Geshe Thupten Junpa. Boston: Wisdom Publications, 2002.

Hanh, Thich Nhat. *Calming The Fearful Mind.* Berkeley: Parallax Press, 2005.

Helminski, Edmund, trans. *The Ruins of the Heart: Selected Lyric Poetry of Jelaluddin Rumi.* Putney, VT: Threshold Books, 1981.

Hixon, Lex. *Great Swan: Meetings with Ramakrishna.* Boston: Shambhala Publications, Inc., 1992.

_____. *Mother of the Universe.* Wheaton, IL: The Theosophical Publishing House, 1994.

Huxley, Aldous. *The Perennial Philosophy.* New York: Harper Colophon, 1970.

Isherwood, Christopher, ed. *Vedanta for the Western World.* New York: The Marcel Rodd Company, 1946.

Jung, C. G. *Psychological Commentary on Kundalini Yoga, Lectures 1 & 2, 1932.* New York: Spring Publications, 1975.

_____. *Aion.* Princeton: Princeton University Press, 1978.

_____. *Symbols of Transformation.* Princeton: Princeton University Press, 1990.

_____. *The Archetypes and The Collective Unconscious.* Princeton: Princeton University Press, 1990.

Kabat-Zinn, Jon. *Wherever You Go There You Are: Mindfulness Meditation In Everyday Life.* New York: Hyperion, 1994.

Kornfield, Jack. *A Path With Heart: A Guide Through the Perils and Promises of Spiritual Life.* New York: Bantam Books, 1993.

Kuhn, Thomas. *The Structure of Scientific Revolutions,* 2nd ed. Chicago, IL: Chicago University Press, 1970.

Kushner, Lawrence. *Eyes Remade For Wonder.* Woodstock, VT: Jewish Lights Publishing, 1998.

Lawrence, Brother. *The Practice of the Presence of God.* Boston: Shambhala, 2005.

Madhavananda, Swami, trans. *Vivekachudamani.* Calcutta, India: Advaita Ashrama, 1982.

Maull, Fleet. *Dharma In Hell: The Prison Writings of Fleet Maull.* Boulder, CO: Prison Dharma Network, 2005.

Merton, Thomas. *The Wisdom of the Desert.* New York: New Directions Publishing Corp., 1960.

Moore, Robert and Douglas Gillette. *King, Warrior, Magician, Lover: Rediscovering the Archetypes of the Mature Masculine.* San Francisco: Harper San Francisco, 1991.

_____. *The King Within.* New York: William Morrow and Co., Inc., 1992.

Muktananda, Swami. *Play of Consciousness.* San Francisco: Harper and Row, 1978.

_____. *Kundalini: The Secret of Life.* South Fallsburg, NY: SYDA Foundation, 1979.

_____. *Kundalini Stavaha.* South Fallsburg, NY: SYDA Foundation, 1980.

Nisargadatta; Maurice Frydman, trans. *I Am That.* Edited by Sudhakar Diskshit. Durham, NC: Acorn Press, 2012.

Pandit, M. P., trans. *Kularnava Tantra.* Madras, India: Ganesh & Co., 1973.

Pearce, Joseph Chilton. *Evolution's End: Claiming the Potential of Our Intelligence.* San Francisco: Harper, 1992.

_____. *The Biology of Transcendence: A Blueprint of the Human Spirit.* Rochester, VT: Park Street Press, 2002.

Perera, Sylvia Brinton. *Descent to the Goddess.* Toronto: Inner City Books, 1981.

Prabhavananda, Swami. "What Yoga Is." In *Vedanta for the Western World,* edited by Christopher Isherwood, 41–46. New York: The Marcel Rodd Company, 1946.

____. "The Goal of Yoga." In *Vedanta for the Western World,* edited by Christopher Isherwood, 47–50. New York: The Marcel Rodd Company, 1946.

____. *How to Know God: The Yoga Aphorisms of Patanjali.* Hollywood, CA: Vedanta Press, 1969.

____. *The Song of God: Bhagavad Gita,* translated by Christopher Isherwood. Hollywood, CA: Vedanta Press, 1972.

____. *Shankara's Crest-jewel of Discrimination,* translated by Christopher Isherwood. Hollywood, CA: Vedanta Press, 1978.

____. *The Upanishads: Breath of the Eternal,* translated by F. Manchester. Hollywood, CA: Vedanta Press, 1957.

Radhakrishnan, S., trans. *The Principal Upanishads.* New York: Humanities Press, 1978.

Rinpoche, Bokar. *Tara: The Feminine Divine.* San Francisco: ClearPoint Press, 1999.

Sasaki, Sokei-an. *Original Nature: Zen Comments on the Sixth Patriarch's Platform Sutra.* Bloomington: iUniverse, 2012.

Schwartz, Jeffrey and Sharon Begley. *The Mind & The Brain: Neuroplasticity and the Power of Mental Force.* New York: Harper Perennial, 2002.

Shaw, Miranda. *Passionate Enlightenment: Women in Tantric Buddhism.* Princeton: Princeton University Press, 1994.

Siegel, Daniel. *Mindsight: The New Science of Personal Transformation.* New York: Bantam Books, 2010.

Silburn, Lilian. *Kundalini: Energy of the Depths.* Albany, NY: SUNY Press, 1988.

Simmer-Brown, Judith. *Dakini's Warm Breath: The Feminine Principle in Tibetan Buddhism.* Boston: Shambhala, 2001.

Singh, Jaideva, trans. *Shiva Sutras.* Delhi, India: Motilal Banarsidass, 1979.

____, trans. *Vijnanabhairava.* Delhi, India: Motilal Banarsidass, 1979.

____, trans. *Spanda-Karikas.* Delhi, India: Motilal Banarsidass, 1980.

_____, trans. *Pratyabhijnahrdayam: The Secret of Self-Recognition*. Delhi, India: Motilal Banarsidass, 1980.

Subramanian, V. K. *Saundaryalahari of Sankaracarya*. Delhi, India: Motilal Banarsidass, 1980.

Sutich, A. "Transpersonal Therapy." *Journal of Transpersonal Psychology*, 5 (1973): 1–6.

Suzuki, Shunryu. *Zen Mind, Beginner's Mind*. New York: Weatherhill, 1975.

SYDA Foundation. *The Nectar of Chanting*. South Fallsburg, NY: SYDA Foundation, 1984.

Taimni, I. K., trans. *The Science of Yoga: The Yoga Sutras of Patanjali*. Wheaton, IL: The Theosophical Publishing House, 1975.

Tart, Charles, ed. *Transpersonal Psychologies*. London: Routledge & Kegan Paul, 1975.

Tigunait, Pandit Rajmani. *Tantra Unveiled*. Honesdale, PA: Himalayan Institute, 2007.

Tirtha, Swami Vishnu. *Devatma Shakti*. Delhi, India: Swami Shivom Tirth, 1974.

Trungpa, Chögyam. *The Collected Works of Chögyam Trungpa, Volume 3: Cutting Through Spiritual Materialism – The Myth Of Freedom – The Heart Of The Buddha – Selected Writings*, edited by Carol Gimian. Boston: Shambhala, 2004.

Trungpa, Chögyam and Francesca Fremantle. *The Tibetan Book of the Dead: The Great Liberation Through Hearing In The Bardo*. Boston: Shambhala, 2003.

Vahia, N. S. et al. "Psychophysiologic Therapy Based on the Concepts of Patanjali." *American Journal of Psychotherapy*, 27 (1972): 557–65.

Venkatesananda, Swami, trans. *The Concise Yoga Vasishtha*. Albany, New York: SUNY Press, 1984.

Walsh, Roger. "The Consciousness Disciplines and the Behavioral Sciences: Questions of Comparison and Assessment." *American Journal of Psychiatry*, 137 (1980): 663–73.

_____. "Meditation Practice and Research." *Journal of Humanistic Psychology*, 23 (1983): 18–50.

Walsh, Roger and Deane Shapiro, eds. *Beyond Health and Normality: Explorations of Exceptional Psychological Well-Being*. New York: Van Nostrand Reinhold, 1983.

Walsh, Roger and Frances Vaughan, eds. *Beyond Ego: Transpersonal Dimensions in Psychology.* Los Angeles, CA: J. P. Tarcher, 1980.

Way, Robert. *The Wisdom of the English Mystics.* New York: New Directions Publishing Corp., 1978.

Welwood, John. *Toward a Psychology of Awakening.* Boston: Shambhala, 2002.

White, John, ed. *Kundalini: Evolution and Enlightenment.* New York: Anchor Books, 1979.

Wilber, Ken. *Integral Psychology.* Boston: Shambhala, 2000.

____. *A Theory of Everything.* Boston: Shambhala, 2000.

Wilson, Stephen. "In Pursuit of Energy: Spiritual Growth in a Yoga Ashram." *Journal of Humanistic Psychology,* 22 (1982): 43–55.

____. "Becoming a Yogi: Resocialization and Deconditioning as Conversion Processes." *Sociological Analysis* 45 (1984): 301–14.

____. "Therapeutic Processes in a Yoga Ashram." *American Journal of Psychotherapy,* 34 (1985): 253–62.

Woodroffe, Sir John, trans. *Tantra of the Great Liberation: Mahanirvana Tantra.* New York: Dover, 1972.

____. *The Serpent Power.* Madras, India: Ganesh and Co., 1973.

____. *The Garland of Letters: Studies in the Mantra-Shastra.* Madras, India: Ganesh & Co., 1974.

____. *Shakti and Shakta.* New York: Dover Publications, 1978.

____. *Principles of Tantra,* Vols. 1–2. Madras, India: Ganesh & Co., 1978.

____. *Introduction to Tantra Shastra.* Madras, India: Ganesh & Co., 1980.

Yogananda, Paramahansa. *Autobiography of a Yogi.* Los Angeles: Self-Realization Fellowship, 2000.

About the Author

Through professional accomplishments in psychology and a lifelong commitment to meditative disciplines, Lawrence Edwards has cultivated a unique perspective that bridges scientific and mystical domains of direct knowledge. As the founder and director of Anam Cara, Inc., a nonprofit educational organization dedicated to teaching meditative practices from a variety of traditions, Dr. Edwards has taught at universities, hospitals, corporations, professional meetings, prisons, hospice programs, and yoga and meditation centers in the US, Canada, and India. He has been the Integrative Care Clinic program manager at the world-renowned Cincinnati Children's Hospital, president of the Northeast Regional Biofeedback Society, president of the Kundalini Research Network, an adjunct faculty member of New York Medical College since 1998, and vice president of a private Jungian psychiatric treatment center where he also taught yoga and meditation.

Dr. Edwards has written numerous books and articles on Kundalini, meditation, and biofeedback. His first book, *The Soul's Journey: Guidance from the Divine Within,* focuses on how Kundalini guides spiritual development from within. His collection of poetry, *Kali's Bazaar,* reflects the deep mystical wisdom that comes through Kundalini's grace. And his audio program, *Awakening Kundalini: The Path to Radical Freedom,* offers guided practices and lectures that summarize a lifetime of study and experience.

About Sounds True

Sounds True is a multimedia publisher whose mission is to inspire and support personal transformation and spiritual awakening. Founded in 1985 and located in Boulder, Colorado, we work with many of the leading spiritual teachers, thinkers, healers, and visionary artists of our time. We strive with every title to preserve the essential "living wisdom" of the author or artist. It is our goal to create products that not only provide information to a reader or listener, but that also embody the quality of a wisdom transmission.

For those seeking genuine transformation, Sounds True is your trusted partner. At SoundsTrue.com you will find a wealth of free resources to support your journey, including exclusive weekly audio interviews, free downloads, interactive learning tools, and other special savings on all our titles.

To learn more, please visit SoundsTrue.com/bonus/free_gifts or call us toll free at 800-333-9185.

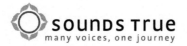

SOUNDS TRUE
many voices, one journey